Praise for
Staying Alive

"Dr. Brenda Hunter has created a roadmap that can assist those dealing with cancer along the path of healing."

—DR. MITCHELL GAYNOR, founder and president,
Gaynor Integrative Oncology

"Finally, a book that goes beyond coping skills for cancer patients! As a breast cancer survivor, I feel empowered to take charge of my own health. *Staying Alive* brings hope to every person who has walked through the dark valley of cancer."

—BECKY HARLING, speaker and author of *A Safe Shelter*

"There is perhaps no more frightening word than *cancer*. For Dr. Brenda Hunter, it was more than a word; it was a diagnosis. In *Staying Alive,* Dr. Hunter walks us through her personal experience in the valley of the shadow of death. She doesn't leave us there, however. By sharing sound strategies that impact body, mind, and spirit, Brenda takes us from hopelessness into healing; from fear into faith."

—JANET PARSHALL, nationally syndicated talk-show host

"Whether you have endured cancer or not, *Staying Alive* gives a game plan for preventative maintenance of your body, emotions, and spirit."

—LINDA DILLOW, author of *Calm My Anxious Heart* and coauthor
of *Intimate Issues*

"A well-written journal on improving your health and staying alive in spite of the complex diagnosis of cancer. [Hunter] has managed to collate the many complex modalities used to treat cancer and has condensed them into pearls of wisdom that would benefit anyone. Plus she gives valuable resources of proven experts for restoring the body, mending the mind, and strengthening our spirits for the battles ahead."

—REX D. RUSSELL, M.D., author of *What the Bible Says
About Healthy Living*

"This fabulous book is a must-read not only for those confronting a cancer diagnosis but also for anyone who wants a healthier, more fulfilled life. Dr. Brenda Hunter has beautifully sifted, sorted, and compiled research and survivors' stories to help us make life-enhancing choices—for mind, body, and spirit."

—LINDA LeSOURD LADER, cofounder, Renaissance Weekends

"I have read Brenda Hunter's *Staying Alive* with intense personal interest since I, too, am a cancer survivor. (I was operated on for a metastasized malignancy at age thirty-six and am now eighty.) Through trial and error I arrived at a few basic lifestyle changes that help keep me healthy. But now Dr. Hunter has found many additional approaches to winning the cancer battle—research that she has laid out in easily accessible and eminently readable form—which I will add to my regimen. What a boon Dr. Hunter's book is to all of us intent on staying alive."

—JOHN SHERRILL, author of *They Speak with Other Tongues*

"Where was this book when we needed it, facing cancer in our family? I suggest that families and spouses read this together, discuss it, argue about all the suggestions on all fronts—physical, emotional and spiritual—put it to work, and see what miracles happen in their own lives."

—LAURAINE SNELLING, author of *The Healing Quilt* and *The Way of Women*

"Dr. Hunter's book is a powerful and practical guide for developing an intentional approach to a healthy lifestyle. Her ideas are as understandable as they are manageable. This book will be an invaluable resource for churches who desire to come alongside those with cancer and to help people live a balanced life, emotionally, physically, and spiritually."

—SUE LANGLIE, Frontline, a ministry of McLean Bible Church, McLean, Virginia

STAYING ALIVE

STAYING
ALIVE

Life-Changing Strategies for Surviving Cancer

RESTORING THE BODY

MENDING THE MIND

STRENGTHENING THE SPIRIT

Brenda Hunter, Ph.D.

FOREWORD BY KEITH I. BLOCK, M.D.

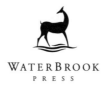

WATERBROOK
PRESS

STAYING ALIVE
PUBLISHED BY WATERBROOK PRESS
2375 Telstar Drive, Suite 160
Colorado Springs, Colorado 80920
A division of Random House, Inc.

This book is based on the author's research and personal and professional experience and has been written to provide insight and encouragement to those with, or concerned about, cancer. None of the information presented in this book is meant to be a prescription for any kind of treatment, medical or otherwise, and reference to organizations and materials is for the reader's convenience only and is not intended as an endorsement. No treatment should be initiated unless recommended and supervised by a qualified professional. In all matters involving health, it is suggested that the reader consult a physician.

Details in some anecdotes and stories have been changed to protect the identities of the persons involved.

Grateful acknowledgment is made to all contributors, in particular for use of material from the following:

The Gerson Therapy. Copyright © 2001 by Dr. Morton Walker and The Gerson Institute. Published by arrangement with Kensington Publishing Corp. All rights reserved. Reprinted by permission of Citadel Press / Kensington Publishing Corp. www.kensingtonbooks.com.

Herbal Medicine, Healing and Cancer: A Comprehensive Program for Prevention and Treatment by D. Yance and A. Valentine, © 1999 Keats Publishing, reprinted by permission of The McGraw-Hill Companies.

ISBN 1-57856-132-9

Copyright © 2004 by Brenda Hunter, Ph.D.

Library of Congress Cataloging-in-Publication Data

Hunter, Brenda.
    Staying alive : life-changing strategies for surviving cancer / Brenda Hunter.— 1st ed.
      p. cm.
Includes bibliographical references.
    ISBN 1-57856-132-9
    1. Cancer—Patients—Rehabilitation. 2. Cancer—Diet therapy. 3. Cancer—Psychological aspects.
4. Cancer—Religious aspects—Christianity. I. Title.
    RC261.H85 2004
    616.99′406—dc22

                                                                                    2003020823

Printed in the United States of America
2004—First Edition

10 9 8 7 6 5 4 3 2 1

. . . . ❖ . . . .

I DEDICATE THIS BOOK TO DR. AHMAD SHAMIM.

He not only strengthened my belief that I could get well,
but he graciously taught me how.

For me, he is and will always be "Dr. Hope."

. . . . ❖ . . . .

CONTENTS

FOREWORD

A cancer diagnosis is a sudden and unexpected event that unleashes a torrent of fear and confusion. It evokes a degree of shock for which patients and their loved ones are wholly unprepared. Those patients who have successfully navigated the many challenges posed by the diagnosis are doing a tremendous service to others by documenting their personal battles—their difficulties as well as their triumphs. Self-reports that lead to recovery provide much needed hope for those who have been recently diagnosed. These reports often encourage new ways of thinking about overcoming a disease that continues to thwart even the most powerful tools of conventional oncology.

Brenda Hunter, Ph.D., first came through the Block Center for Integrative Cancer Care in 1998 after reading about our approach in a book on alternative cancer treatment options. She had been battling her disease for a short period of time. A woman of strong conviction, she affirmed a deep desire to be an active agent in her own care. It was also her hope that the treatment plan I laid out for her would preclude highly invasive or toxic treatments that could be harmful to her self-healing resources.

Brenda immediately felt reassured with my philosophy of care. She felt a strong affinity with a principle I had championed, called "medical gradualism." According to this principle, physicians should generally look to the least invasive forms of treatment before considering the more invasive or aggressive forms. She also appreciated our emphasis on treating each patient as an integrated whole, promoting a fusion of body and biology, mind and spirit, nutrients and drugs—again, using the latter only after careful consideration of the medical circumstances.

For more than two decades, my colleagues and I have studied the important interconnected role of therapeutic nutrition, exercise physiology, mind-body stress care, and advanced body-centered therapies in the full healing process. Our approach judiciously couples conventional treatment protocols with innovative and integrative strategies that are designed to maximize the treatment benefits while minimizing possible side effects. As Brenda understood early on, our approach is grounded in the tenet that the best medical care is highly individualized through precise clinical and laboratory assessments aimed at specifically bolstering each patient's biological, physical, emotional, and spiritual resources.

Fortunately, Brenda was able to avoid chemotherapy and other more invasive medical treatments. But even in advanced cancer cases for which these treatments may be necessary, it is possible to mitigate toxicity with circadian timing of chemotherapy and with natural agents that promote detoxification and selectively protect normal tissues. Our preliminary data from studies of advanced breast and prostate cancer, soon to be published in peer-review journals, have demonstrated the power of this approach. It is also clear, as Brenda's own case demonstrates, that different levels of disease do indeed warrant different levels of intervention—and that sometimes the softer treatment path is indeed the most appropriate.

Brenda wrote *Staying Alive* after making many substantial changes in her diet, work habits, lifestyle, and outlook. She has combined her training in psychology with her ability to authentically empathize with those facing cancer. This unique fusion enables her to offer light to those in a dark place—and to hold on to that light throughout this deeply personal ordeal. I believe her book will inspire people with cancer to live full and meaningful lives and empower them to more actively participate in the efforts to beat their disease.

In a very real sense, the true experts on the cancer experience are those who have faced the disease themselves. As a psychologist and cancer survivor, Brenda knows that some of the most critical information on survivorship is best revealed by self-report. Her own recovery process, as reflected in the tone and content of these pages, has been continually impelled by her deep reserves of courage, stamina, and faith. She also has constructed an exemplary support team that includes her husband, family, friends, and integrated medical guides.

Throughout this book, Brenda reinforces her own firsthand experiences and insights with those of other survivors she interviewed. The author then balances these personal accounts with perspectives from experts in the fields of nutrition and cancer medicine. The result is a compendium of useful information for anyone struggling with cancer and should be helpful to families and friends of cancer patients. Dr. Hunter's survival story provides a road map of therapeutic possibility for those interested in a more holistic approach, for those who need to feel more fully supported along the journey to an enduring recovery.

KEITH I. BLOCK, M.D.
www.BlockMD.com

KEITH I. BLOCK, M.D., is the Medical and Scientific Director of Block Center for Integrative Cancer Care; Editor-in-Chief of *Integrative Cancer Therapies*, Sage Science Press; Clinical Assistant Professor, University of Illinois College of Medicine at Chicago; Adjunct Assistant Professor of Pharmacognosy, College of Pharmacy, University of Illinois at Chicago; and Medical Consultant on Nutritional-Oncology Research for the Office of Technology Assessment for the Congress of the United States.

ACKNOWLEDGMENTS

Writing this book has been a stimulating, exhausting, and profound experience. I have ventured into areas in which I have no mastery, like nutrition and medicine, and where I have had to rely on the experts—those knowledgeable and dedicated physicians, nutritionists, and psychologists who work with cancer patients. Those I approached were not only willing to grant interviews but in the final days, to fax answers to my follow-up questions. I heard from both Dr. Keith Block and Dr. Nicholas Gonzalez during those frantic last two days of writing as they attempted to answer my questions between consultations with their patients. How's that for helping a writer meet her deadline!

I offer my sincere thanks to all those physicians willing to be interviewed and to share their expertise with the readers of this book. My thanks to Dr. Keith Block, Dr. Mitchell Gaynor, Dr. Nicholas Gonzalez, Dr. James Gordon, Dr. Harold Koenig, Dr. Robert Maunder, Dr. Dean Ornish, Dr. Rex Russell, and Dr. Ahmad Shamim. I am especially grateful that Dr. Gonzalez took the time to read my chapter on detoxification and that Dr. Block and Dr. Shamim read the chapters on detoxification and nutrition. I can sleep better at night knowing those chapters were vetted by these cancer docs.

In addition, I was excited to hear firsthand from Lilian Thompson, Ph.D., at the University of Toronto Medical School, about her research on flaxseed and breast cancer. What I learned from her only solidified my conviction that flaxseed is a miracle food, particularly for those who have had breast cancer.

As for psychologists I interviewed, I am indebted to Dr. Ruth Bollentino, Dr. Gary Cobb, Dr. Shirley Taffel, and Dr. Lydia Temoshok for taking the time to talk with me about their intensive work with cancer patients. And how can I ever express what Dr. Gary Cobb and psychotherapist Dorothy Firman meant to me on a deeply personal level as I sought their help in healing my emotions and my life.

In addition, I want to thank Brian and Anna Maria Clement for the wonderful week at Hippocrates in West Palm Beach, which inspired a chapter in this book. When I called and asked if I could come and learn about the work they are doing, they responded emphatically, "Come." This husband-wife team is not only smart and articulate but beautifully suited for the work they do in educating people on how to reclaim their health through diet.

Since I never intended to write a book containing just interviews with the experts, I went looking for those courageous, resilient individuals who had struggled with cancer years earlier but who today are living rich and rewarding lives. My thanks to all of you for sharing your stories with me and the readers of this book. Since some of you preferred to remain anonymous, I won't list you by name, but I want each of you to know I was moved and inspired by your fight to stay alive, and I believe others will be as well.

When my editor, Carol Bartley, suggested it would help readers to have some tasty vegetarian recipes included in the book, I immediately called the Hippocrates Institute and my two favorite restaurants, The Manatee Café in old St. Augustine, Florida, and The Laughing Seed Café in Asheville, North Carolina. My thanks and appreciation go to Executive Chef Kelly Serbonich at Hippocrates Institute, Executive Chef Cheryl Crosley at The Manatee Café, and Executive Chef Joan Eckert of The Laughing Seed for your willingness to share some of your delicious recipes with readers. In addition, I wish to thank Penny Block for allowing me to include recipes from her book, *A Banquet of Health,* which are based on Dr. Keith Block's patented nutritional program.

I am enormously grateful to my husband, Don, who gave practical and emotional support during the writing of this book as he did for all the others. As crunch time came, he took over the job of obtaining the legal permissions and willingly became my assistant, faxing forms, talking to my editor and contacts at various publishers. We were a team during those last, stressful, mad days of rushing to finish this book. Don, you are my number one cheerleader! Thank you.

My daughter Holly also deserves my thanks and appreciation. She came on board at a critical time to help with the editing, writing, and word processing. An excellent writer, a computer whiz, and a fine editor, Holly gave me rich and essential help.

Finally, abundant thanks and appreciation to my editor and friend, Carol Bartley. I specifically asked Laura Barker, the editorial director at WaterBrook, if I could work with Carol on this book, not only because I had worked with her on three previous ones, but also because Carol is a warm, empathic, smart woman and an exacting editor who asks hard questions and sends me back to rethink and rewrite, again and again. Now, I wasn't always happy about this, but the book is better for it. Carol—I mean this—the book would not have been written without your help. It's the toughest book I've ever written, and when I would, on occasion, call you to whine, you invariably made me laugh! In the end we were both working and faxing like mad women. Thank you, Carol, for your friendship, excellent editorial help, and canny advice. Truly, you helped me create this book. You joined me in believing that this book could inspire and aid those struggling with cancer. What a gift. Thank you. Now we both need a vacation!

ENTERING THE CANCER ZONE

There is in the worst of fortunes the best of chances for a happy change.
EURIPIDES

God who sends the wound, sends the medicine.
CERVANTES

It was well after eleven o'clock on a chilly Good Friday night. My husband and I had gone to church earlier that evening, and now I was battling my usual insomnia while Don snored gently beside me. He made soft, intermittent *whoozing* sounds that irritated me. As I struggled to find a comfortable position in bed, I rolled over on my right side and for no apparent reason slid my hand along the contour of my right breast where I felt a...*lump?* Could it be? Impossible! Instantly my mind went on red alert. I sat up, adrenaline coursing through my body, lifted my nightshirt, and retraced the contour of my breast with trembling fingers. Yes, there it was—a hard, movable lump bigger than a dime but smaller than a quarter.

With mounting fear I shook my husband awake. "Don, please, please wake up. I think I've found a lump in my breast. Can you feel it?"

Still sleepy, Don touched my breast, hesitated, and then said quietly, "Yes, I feel a lump."

My mind raced toward my worst fear. *Breast cancer.* Suddenly I realized it was the weekend; I wouldn't be able to see my gynecologist for two days. Two whole days of not knowing. Two whole days of suspecting the worst.

Attempting to comfort me, Don said reassuringly, "You know, Brenda, this may not be serious. Aren't most breast lumps benign?"

I listened but refused to be comforted. I'd never found a lump in my breast before, but the previous year I had been called back after a mammogram had revealed a thickening in that same area of my right breast. When I remembered *that* piece of data, I moaned. I just knew it was cancer. My husband put his arms around me tenderly, quietly prayed that I would be okay, and eventually dropped off to sleep.

I lay awake until dawn.

The weekend crawled by. My mother was with us for the Easter holiday, visiting from her nursing home in North Carolina. Because she was struggling with serious illness herself and was not a particularly empathic listener, I decided not to tell her about the lump. I also decided not to tell my daughters until I had seen my gynecologist. Why alarm them unnecessarily? So Don and I went through the motions of a normal family holiday with Mother and our grown children. It was excruciating. I tried to control my fearful thoughts and mounting anxiety as I prepared meals, took Mother shopping, and sat in church on Easter morning, yet my mind was anywhere but the present. I waited impatiently for Monday, sending short, terse prayers heavenward. *Please, God, don't let me have breast cancer! Please, God!*

When Monday morning finally arrived, I bolted out of bed, showered, dressed, and hastily bid my mother good-bye. Don and I had agreed he would take her back to North Carolina and call me in late afternoon. As I heard the last car door slam, I dashed for the phone and started dialing my gynecologist's office. No answer. After dialing repeatedly, I finally got the receptionist, and within an hour I was sitting on the edge of the examining table, nervously clutching my white paper gown. Since my doctor was away on vacation, I was being seen by her partner, a woman I'd never met.

As I waited impatiently, I scanned the examining room for a magazine, a telephone book—anything to distract me. Nothing. Just sterile white walls, an examining table, and a single chair on which I had draped my clothes. The longer I waited, the more desperate I felt. *Please, God, have the doctor come quickly and let her give me hope.* When the door opened, a tall, slender woman clad in a white lab coat with a stethoscope draped around her neck entered. "Hi," she said cheerfully. "How're you doing?" Without waiting for an answer, she continued, "The nurse said you found a lump in your right breast over the weekend. Is that right?" When I nodded yes, she said, "Let's take a look."

The doctor bent over me. Her hands moved efficiently around the surface of my right breast, pausing to finger the lump, and then she thrust her fingers into the pit of my right arm. I lay perfectly still on the examining table, trying to pray, as the doctor moved to my left breast, repeating the ritual. Then she stood upright and waited for me to sit up. With a matter-of-fact tone of voice, she said, "Well, you have a hard, movable lump in your right breast. It's probably malignant, and when a tumor is this large, it has usually metastasized throughout the body."

I was stunned. My anxiety exploded into terror. From breast cancer to metastasized cancer? From a shot at survival to a certain death sentence? How could this have happened? I heard a roar in my ears and felt as if I were plunging into an abyss. My mouth dry, I tentatively asked the doctor a few questions, hoping for some reassurance or empathy. But I hoped in vain. The doctor headed quickly toward the door. "I'll call to get you in to see a radiologist this afternoon," she said as she sailed out of the room.

With a heavy heart, I dressed quickly and took the elevator down several floors. My heart was thumping wildly, and I could feel a migraine forming in the back of my skull. I had been so anxious at breakfast I hadn't eaten anything.

As I left the building and gazed at the blue sky, I realized I had never felt so utterly alone or devastated in my life. Then I reached my car, where to my chagrin I found a yellow parking ticket tucked under my windshield wiper. Unlocking the door, I fell onto the front seat, sobbing.

Within hours I was at a radiology center having a mammogram. The radiologist, while openly angry with the gynecologist for pronouncing a premature death sentence, reluctantly gave me his own bleak diagnosis. "I'm sorry to say this, but the lump is probably malignant. However, no one knows at this point if the cancer has spread to your lymph nodes." Visibly uncomfortable, he offered me a thin shard of hope. "Just be glad your lump is movable." When I asked what he meant, he said that an immovable lump would mean it was attached to the chest wall and the cancer had most likely invaded my lung, resulting in an even worse prognosis.

I went out to the waiting room, where my lovely and very pregnant daughter Kristen anxiously sat, pretending to read a magazine. I told her my news, and we walked slowly back to the car. Kristen drove me home, trying to find words to comfort me. I listened distractedly, feeling all the while as if a heat-seeking missile had just blasted my torso.

An hour later Don called from North Carolina, and I told him what the two doctors had said. Shocked, he said quietly, "Don't forget, we're in this together. I'm coming right home and will be there by midnight."

That night I made myself a salad but couldn't taste the food. Afterward I sat on the living room sofa, numbly staring out into the black, implacable night. As I sat there, it occurred to me that life as I had known it was over. No more once-a-year physicals. No more easy reliance on good health. For starters, I needed to find a surgeon. Pronto. He would then refer me to an oncologist and a radiologist if necessary. *Oncologist? Radiologist?* Now these were scary words. Didn't oncologists treat cancer patients with toxic drugs that made them throw up and lose their hair? And I didn't like the visual image that the word *radiologist* conjured up—I could see myself lying on a cold metal examining table as invisible radioactive beams penetrated my breast. Slowly it dawned on me that I would be shuttled among a growing number of doctors in the immediate future, and yet it might be weeks before I knew what was going on in my body. Weeks of fear and anxiety with no respite in sight.

Finally I heard Don's car crunching up our gravel driveway. When he came in the door, I walked toward him. No words, just tears. We held each other, talked briefly, and fell into bed, wasted by the trauma of the day. While Don quickly fell asleep, my mind replayed the events and words of the day over and over. Against my will and to my absolute horror, I was entering a new land filled with eerie shadows, images of death, and dire pronouncements delivered by doctors I did not know and had never wanted to meet. A territory where I had neither a map nor a guide. A place I had no guarantee of leaving alive. The Cancer Zone.

THE CANCER ZONE

Within days I had selected a surgeon reputed to be one of the best breast surgeons in the northern Virginia area. A short, stocky Spaniard, Dr. Ortega[1] introduced himself, took my hand, and led me into the examining room. He seemed genuinely warm and friendly and was obviously used to reassuring frightened women who appeared at his office carrying x-rays in official-looking Manila envelopes. After he had looked at my x-rays of the scary white tumor with its hairy edges, Dr. Ortega dashed my last hope that the tumor was benign by casually saying, "I've examined lots of x-rays during the past twenty years, and I think this tumor is probably malignant."

Then he turned to me and said, "Let me examine you." After the breast exam, Dr. Ortega announced in his charming accent, "Even though you probably have breast cancer, you'll be just fine." *Just fine?* How could these two ideas logically coexist? When he saw the look of disbelief on my face, he explained, "I don't believe the cancer has spread to your lymph nodes." Although I knew almost nothing about cancer's relentless march through the body, I intuited that this was good news. Finally some comfort. "Get my nurse to schedule surgery, and then we'll know for sure," he said as he turned to go. Dr. Ortega was so convinced the tumor was malignant that he wanted to skip the biopsy and immediately remove the lump.

Within days Dr. Ortega had removed the lump, and the pathology report confirmed his conviction that it was indeed malignant. After delivering the bad news, the doctor told me he would need to operate again since he didn't get clean margins the first time, and cancer cells still lurked in my breast tissue. Besides, he wanted to remove fifteen lymph nodes to see if the cancer had metastasized. My options were to get the equivalent of a lumpectomy plus radiation or a full mastectomy. So I could better understand the choices that horrified me, Dr. Ortega sent me to a Harvard-educated radiologist he recommended.

The visit with the radiologist did not go well. When she told me that radiating my right breast would damage a portion of my right lung, possibly causing a secondary cancer in the years to come, I yelped, "But what if I live another twenty years and need two healthy lungs?" The look on her face told me she didn't expect me to live that long.

With a heavy heart, I realized I needed to make some life-and-death decisions. And fast. Wanting to lessen the risk of a secondary cancer, I decided to have a mastectomy and forgo radiation altogether. It mattered enormously that I had two good friends who were long-term breast-cancer survivors, and both had undergone mastectomies. Not having the heart to research the pros and cons of mastectomies versus lumpectomies, I went with my gut even though Dr. Ortega advised me to have a lumpectomy and radiation. Unhappy with my decision, he reluctantly agreed to perform the mastectomy. What he didn't understand was that ultimately emotion had triumphed over reason. The fact that research showed a lumpectomy plus radiation was as effective as a mastectomy alone and a whole lot less disfiguring didn't matter to me. What mattered was that my friends had chosen mastectomies, and *they were still alive!*

Hey, staying alive was what I was about. Yet when the time came to actually have my breast removed, I didn't feel brave or cocky at all. As I lay on the gurney waiting to be wheeled up to surgery, I wanted to jump up, rip off the surgical gown, and run. Run as fast as I could. Anywhere. Away from the hospital and my life. Away from *me*—from the body that had, after years of excellent health, betrayed me.

The minutes ticked by on the clock overhead. It was seven o'clock on a Friday night. I had chosen to have surgery on this particular night so that Dr. Greenman, who had assisted Dr. Ortega during the first surgery, could be my anesthesiologist. I had even called the anesthesiology department to see when he was on call. He had cheered me up weeks earlier, and since I was afraid of undergoing general anesthesia, I wanted his comforting, lighthearted presence. Soon Dr. Greenman appeared. As he inserted the needle into the vein in my left arm, I said half mockingly, half seriously, "I'm not going to die tonight, am I?"

He looked down at me and said with a smile, "I *hate it* when people do that! If you do, I'll never speak to you again." I laughed and caught the plastic cap he tossed me as he walked away.

Later Dr. Ortega told me that Dr. Greenman had had a schedule change and was not supposed to work that night. But when the hospital nurse told him that I was counting on him, he called his wife to say he would be late, that he was going to assist in one more surgery. Mine. It still makes me happy to remember the kindness of this man who worked on a Friday night when he didn't have to.

You can't imagine how grateful I was to wake up! I was still alive, although I had drains descending from my right armpit, and my chest was swathed in bandages. All that night a nurse monitored my vital signs, and the next day Dr. Ortega came to examine the incision. "Beautiful," he said as I nervously looked out the window.

While I was grateful to have the surgeries behind me, I had greatly underestimated the profound psychological impact of losing a breast. As with many women, my breasts represented a significant part of my body image, my femininity, my sexuality. Now one of mine was gone, and I wondered how that would affect my feelings about myself as a woman. And how would my husband respond to a single-breasted wife?

In the days ahead, when I needed to cleanse the wound in the shower, I closed my eyes, let the warm water do its magic, and waited, averting my eyes, while Don tenderly toweled me dry. When I went to the surgeon for my first visit after surgery, he asked, "Who's taking care of your incision?"

"My husband," I said. "I'm not ready to look at it yet."

"He's a good man," responded Dr. Ortega.

I nodded. So he was and is.

The Sunday I came home from the hospital, the reality of what I'd chosen to do washed over me. Every time I moved, the drains pulled on tender skin. They reminded me that I had not only lost a breast but had also had fifteen lymph nodes excised. I was physically weaker than I could ever remember. In addition, I felt disfigured. As I lay on my bed, spent from the exertion of coming home, my compassionate daughters climbed onto the bed with me, one on each side. As they took my hands, I started to cry. "I feel so sad that I've lost my breast," I sobbed. Tender and solicitous, my children assured me that it would not matter someday. They were right, but on that day and for days afterward, I mourned my loss.

Hours later when I checked our phone messages, I heard my dear friend Carlie's voice: "Brenda, I know today will be especially hard for you. You're probably just beginning to come to terms emotionally with what it means to lose a breast. But I want you to know that everything that's important about you is still intact."

Intact. I felt anything but intact that black Sunday. But even in my suffering, I was moved by Carlie's words as well as her keen insight and kindness. I saved her message as long as possible, replaying it again and again.

CUT, POISON, AND BURN

Soon after the mastectomy, Dr. Ortega told me he had been wrong, that the cancer had spread to one of my lymph nodes. How quickly this changed both my prognosis and my mental outlook. Because the cancer had metastasized, Dr. Ortega no longer said I would be "just fine"; instead he said soberly that if I followed the protocol the oncologist recommended, I would increase my chances of surviving to the ten-year mark. With a heavy heart, I made an appointment with the oncologist to discuss treatment plans.

As you probably know, a visit to an oncologist is one of the scariest things on earth, easily akin to boarding a plane immediately after a terrorist attack. I noticed, as I sat in this doctor's waiting room, that those who had come for chemotherapy treatments looked anxious and scared. In fact, an elderly woman next to me was audibly hyperventilating as she waited for her name to be called.

When the nurse finally said, "Dr. Hunter," I walked toward Dr. Blake's[2] office, sat down, and listened as the bespectacled, forty-something oncologist calmly told me my statistical chances of recurrence, depending on which treatment option I chose. Looking up from the pathology report, he said, "Because you had one malignant node, you have a 50 percent chance of recurrence in the next ten years. Yours is considered stage 2 breast cancer." He went on to discuss the size of the tumor (two centimeters) and its level of aggressiveness (slow growing). As I listened, I struggled to understand this new medical vocabulary and my statistical odds of survival. Although I had studied statistics at Georgetown University, these current stats held a whole new meaning. With a growing feeling of nausea, I thought, *These are my death statistics.*

Just when I thought I couldn't bear any more bad news, Dr. Blake recommended that I take Adriamycin, a chemotherapy drug so toxic it could damage my heart. My heart! I had already lost a breast; I certainly didn't want to damage my heart! My heart was functioning just fine, thank you. Why, I wondered, did the cure sound as bad as the disease?

When I left the oncologist's office that day, I knew I needed help. The past several weeks had been incredibly draining, emotionally and physically. Conventional medicine's "cut, poison, and burn" approach to cancer just didn't make sense to me. Why take a sick body with a depressed immune system and subject it to a treatment protocol that might damage vital organs and cause secondary cancers? Frankly, the "cure" sounded barbaric. While I knew that doing nothing was not an option, the treatment protocols I had heard so far gave me little confidence. I longed for a treatment plan that would end the abnormal proliferation of cancer cells, strengthen my immune system, and give me a fighting chance for survival. Did such a plan even exist? Also, I needed a doctor who would respect my desire to actively participate in any cancer care and who held out hope that I could beat the disease.

I didn't know it at the time, but I had just discovered my fighting spirit.

A New Ally

The summer before my diagnosis I had taken a graduate course at Johns Hopkins designed to help therapists better understand cancer and its devastating emotional impact. The professor who taught the course, Dr. Linda Seligman, was not only a practicing psychotherapist but also a breast-cancer survivor. Within days of my traumatic visit to the oncologist, I made an appointment to see her. As it turned out, this was one of the best gifts I gave myself during this particularly stressful time. Although I later chose a different road in my cancer journey than she, Dr. Seligman supported me as I made my treatment decisions. "Once somebody gets a cancer diagnosis, the road ahead is uncertain," she said. "It makes sense that your suppressed immune system will function better if you follow a course of treatment you believe in."

What a relief to hear this voice of reason! Moreover, Dr. Seligman validated my feelings and told me that even after seven years she still thinks about cancer every day. She has, however, learned to push her fears aside as she enjoys a busy and rewarding life as both a professor and therapist.

I was grateful for her encouragement to follow my mind and heart in making my treatment decisions. To have been railroaded into a course of action before I was ready would have been psychologically disastrous for me. I needed time to process all the overwhelming data I'd been given. Time to listen to my heart. Time to talk to breast-cancer survivors who had gone before me. Time to pray.

One thing became clear in those troubling and intense early days: Any decisions I made I would have to live with and possibly die with. My goal was not to deny the severity of my illness but to combat it on all fronts: the physical (which was *all* the doctors had discussed so far), the psychological, and the spiritual. To maximize my chances of survival, I desperately needed to believe in the efficacy of any treatment I chose, and it needed to be multifaceted. And if I lost the battle? I wanted no regrets.

What if my family did not agree with my decisions? Then I wanted them to respect my decisions and not try to convince me to take a different path. I had to be wholehearted about any course of action I took, because bringing my body back from its severely weakened condition would take all of my powers. As it turned out, my husband and daughters did not agree with my ultimate decisions. However, they loved me enough to support me and not try to force their opinions on me. For this I will be eternally grateful. As it has turned out, they now feel I made the best decisions for me.

A Ray of Hope

Since I believe in second opinions, Don and I drove to Baltimore, Maryland, to the prestigious teaching hospital Johns Hopkins so I could see an oncologist there. This warm and humane man said he didn't believe chemotherapy was absolutely necessary for me. "The benefits have to outweigh the risks of these highly potent drugs, and your cancer was detected early and was slow growing, and you had only one malignant lymph node." He added, "I wouldn't run after you today if you left the hospital refusing to take chemotherapy, but I would if you refused to take tamoxifen." Then in his genial Irish brogue, the doctor explained the benefits of tamoxifen, the hormonal therapy of choice for those, like me, who are estrogen-receptor positive. After our conversation, I left Hopkins feeling hopeful for the first time since I had been diagnosed.

The Prayer of Jehoshaphat

One morning during this intensely stressful time, Don and I sat at the dining room table, lingering over breakfast. By now I had collected all my statistics, gone for a second opinion, and had even evaluated a meta-analysis of all the American and European tamoxifen studies with my dear friend Chap, a statistician, who had helped me understand the truth behind the numbers. The meta-analysis showed that while tamoxifen reduces the incidence of breast-cancer recurrence, it does not significantly affect survival rates long term. As Dr. John Lee says in *What Your Doctor May Not Tell You About Breast Cancer,* "It has never been shown that tamoxifen reduced the mortality rate of women using it long term, regardless of its protection against breast cancer. In other words, if you use tamoxifen, it may reduce your risk of breast cancer for a while, but there's an approximately equal chance that it will cause you to get something equally serious or to die from something else."[3] Dr. Lee also states that tamoxifen triples the risk of fatal blood clots in the lung, increases the risk of stroke and blindness, and may even cause liver dysfunction.[4]

At that point I was confused and bewildered. What should I do?

On that particular morning Don and I were reading chapter 20 of the Old Testament book of 2 Chronicles. This is the story of good King Jehoshaphat of Judah, who finds himself surrounded by a "vast army" of enemies—the Moabites and Ammonites. Afraid, he assembles all of Judah, including the little ones, to stand before the Lord. Casting himself upon heaven's mercy, the king says to the Lord, "We do not know what to do, but our eyes are upon you" (verse 12).

Everything in me responded to those simple but profound words. I turned to Don and said, "I *don't* know what to do, and talking to the docs and analyzing the data haven't brought me any closer to an answer. Why not pray the prayer of Jehoshaphat?" So we prayed, and in my heart and my mind I, like the ancient king of Judah, cast myself on God's mercy. Within days I heard about a doctor in Laurel, Maryland, who reputedly has kept hundreds of cancer patients alive through an anticancer diet, supplements, and detoxification of the body.

Encouraged by this doctor's reputation and believing this was an answer to prayer, one midsummer morning Don and I drove to see Dr. Ahmad Shamim and discovered that this surgeon-turned-nutritional-therapist believes that a cancer patient's first line of defense lies in enhancing his immune system while at the same time nourishing his malnourished body. He explained to me that even though I was overweight (I had added twenty pounds during my hormone replacement therapy days), the mere fact that I had cancer indicated that my body was not absorbing nutrients well and that my digestion needed improvement. Dr. Shamim believes that detoxifying the body and attending to the gut are hugely important. I left the office of this gentle Iranian, a man I later dubbed "Dr. Hope," with guidelines for a radical dietary change, a list of enzymes, vitamins, minerals, and herbal supplements, and a protocol for detoxifying and cleansing my body. He also prescribed an anticandida (yeast) medication since an overgrowth of yeast, which he believes all cancer patients have, is a powerful enemy of the immune system.

Later I learned from Dr. Shamim that his sister had "died from the treatment" she took to combat cancer and that her suffering had prompted him to learn about nutritional therapies and their effect on the immune system. "Also," Dr. Shamim told me, "I got tired of taking out diseased organs." He added that surgery "did not address the root cause of disease." That fortuitous visit to the good doctor's office occurred nearly six years ago and was the start of a nutritional program that gives me abundant energy, nights of peaceful sleep, and the hope that I can beat cancer.

Based on all I learned during those early weeks, I chose not to take chemotherapy, believing that for me the risks outweighed the benefits. I did go on tamoxifen for a while as I began to implement Dr. Shamim's program to strengthen my immune system. Unfortunately, I became so wired I couldn't sleep, and I was severely depressed on the drug. When I reported these side effects to the oncologist at Johns Hopkins, he said that a small percentage of women can't take tamoxifen because it triggers raging depression. Since quality of life was (and is) important to me, I discontinued the drug and started down a path without signs or markers to guide me, knowing there was no going back.

Scared and conscious of my uncertain future, I put my hand in God's, summoned all the courage I could muster, and forged ahead.

A Holistic Approach to Staying Alive

In the months and years since that fateful Good Friday weekend, I have discovered that cancer is a complex, multifaceted illness with deep roots that extend not only into our bodies but into our minds and spirits as well. We should not just treat our bodies with surgery, powerful drugs, and radiation and expect to get and stay well. We need to change the internal and external terrain of our lives that caused the cancer cells to proliferate with abandon in the first place. Our bodies are highly responsive to chronic stress; the high-fat, processed diet most Americans eat; difficult relationships; unhealed childhood wounds; and the absence of a sense of meaning and purpose. Therefore, *to heal our bodies, we must heal our lives.* The good news is that we have wonderful, self-healing bodies that long to be well, and given the proper tools and right information, many of us can recover our health if we are willing to radically change certain aspects of our lives.

Facing the fiercest battle of my life, I have worked hard to create an integrated approach to cancer care and survival that involves the whole person: body, mind, and spirit. I know how difficult it is to find comprehensive help in those early months when our lives have been upended and we are terrified that we might die. My friend Chip Morgan, a gastroenterologist, told me when he was struggling with lung cancer, "I don't have the inclination or the energy to read a lot of books, but I'd read one book if I thought it could help me address this illness on all fronts."

This book is the result of all that I, as a psychologist, researcher, and six-year cancer survivor, have learned about staying alive and wholeheartedly embracing life after a cancer diagnosis. In writing this book I have interviewed cancer experts like Dr. Keith Block, Dr. Mitchell Gaynor, Dr. Nicholas Gonzalez, Dr. James Gordon, Dr. Dean Ornish, and my own Dr. Ahmad Shamim. I have traveled to the Hippocrates Health Institute in Florida, a place of healing that for fifty years has treated many with catastrophic cancers. In my conversations with physicians and therapists who work with cancer patients, I asked, "What do those who survive this disease have in common?" And I have interviewed long-term cancer survivors, some of whom took all the treatments that conventional medicine had to offer, while others chose a different path. "What," I asked, "helped you to survive?" These success stories will encourage you and challenge you to look at life-changing strategies you can use as you work to reclaim your health.

While this book has been written primarily for those of you struggling with cancer, to help you move beyond fear and confusion to empowerment and hope, it is also designed for those of you who are interested in cancer prevention. Cancer has reached epidemic proportions in this country; experts predict about 1,334,100 new cases of cancer to be diagnosed in 2003.[5] But it is a highly preventable disease, states Dr. Mitchell Gaynor, Director of Medical Oncology at the Strang Cancer Prevention Center in New York City. According to the National Cancer Institute, diet is believed to be the major cause of some 30 to 70 percent of all cancers.[6] And it is well established in the psychological literature that a certain personality type— a giving-till-it-hurts, other-focused personality—is prone to cancer. Moreover, in my interviews I have discovered that cancer patients have usually experienced years of chronic stress before the onset of the disease. They have difficulty nurturing themselves, and they may struggle with a pervasive lack of self-love. If any of this describes you or your life, this book can help you make important changes that will enhance your health and your life.

So let's begin our journey toward self-discovery and healing, learning strategies for preventing and surviving cancer. Where do we begin? We begin by asking an important question: What is cancer saying about our lives? Join me as we look at all the different messages cancer gives us, and learn how different people have responded to cancer, changed their minds and their lives, and survived.

WHAT IS CANCER SAYING ABOUT OUR LIVES?

Sickness is an indication that our way of life is not in harmony with the environment.… If we have cancer, for example, we accept what it has to teach us about ourselves.

MICHIO KUSHI

There is no agony like bearing an untold story inside you.

ZORA NEALE HURSTON

I am sitting with my friend Chip Morgan at a restaurant in downtown Asheville, North Carolina. He and I are having green tea as we talk about something we have in common—a cancer diagnosis. Chip, a warm, engaging father of four, chose to treat his lung cancer with surgery, chemotherapy, and radiation. Today he looks vital and healthy after a recent trip to Wild Dunes, South Carolina, with his family. When I ask him what his greatest concern was after he had made his treatment decisions, he promptly replies, "I asked myself, 'What is cancer saying about my life?'"

Chip's words resonate with me. Shortly after my initial scramble to assemble a medical team and choose a course of treatment, I, too, began to ask myself that question. What message was I to derive from this illness? After all, I hadn't always had cancer. In fact, I had enjoyed excellent health until I reached forty. When I worried about future health problems, I was concerned only about heart disease, the number one killer for women, because I had already lost a father and grandfather to this disease. What had happened in my life to make me vulnerable to cancer at the age of fifty-six? And how could I stave off a recurrence?

The oncologist had already told me I had a high probability of breast-cancer recurrence. When I mentioned this to Dr. Ortega, he said, "From now on, 80 percent of what happens to you will be the result of what occurs above the shoulders." It slowly dawned on me that he was saying our minds and emotions have an enormous impact on the outcome once we receive a cancer diagnosis. Unbeknown to the doctor, his comment was my introduction to the mind-body connection in cancer.

Searching for a Holistic Approach

As I searched for a holistic approach to cancer recovery, I couldn't escape the impression that cancer has conventional medicine stumped. Even with the plethora of cancer drugs on the market—and news analysts herald the advent of a new cancer bullet regularly—cancer is *still* the second leading cause of death in the United States, exceeded only by heart disease. So lethal is it that, according to the American Cancer Society, Americans have a one in four chance of dying of cancer.[1] In fact, in 2003 approximately 556,500 Americans were expected to die of cancer, or more than 1,500 people every day.[2] So cancer rates have skyrocketed in this country despite the war on cancer that President Nixon declared in 1971.

Conventional medicine currently views cancer as a raging cellular disorder and considers cancer "cured" as long as the tumor has been excised, most of the malignant cells killed, and the symptoms alleviated for a period of years; but to me this seems a simplistic view that doesn't take into account the influence of mind, emotions, spirit, and what was happening in the patient's life in the years leading up to cancer. After all, cancer does not just spring up *ex nihilo* in the body but can take decades to develop.

I realized I would have to go far beyond what conventional medicine had to offer if I wanted a multifaceted, holistic approach to cancer recovery. Apparently I am not alone, since *Newsweek* magazine states that roughly half of all Americans look outside conventional medicine for a part of their overall medical care.[3] In fact, Americans spend some $30 billion a year out of their own pockets (with no insurance compensation) for visits to nonconventional healers that include naturopathic physicians, chiropractors, acupuncturists, herbalists, massage therapists, and doctors of Chinese medicine.[4] Complementary and alternative medicine (CAM) is not a single, unified tradition like conventional medicine, yet after almost a hundred years of viewing CAM therapies as downright quackery, many conventionally trained physicians are scrambling to learn about herbs, acupuncture, biofeedback, and nutrition simply because the "public believes in them."[5] Also, since many of their patients are taking herbs along with their prescription medicines, doctors need to understand herbal-drug interactions to advise their patients. And an increasing number of medical schools are offering courses in CAM therapies. Moreover, in recent years, the National Institutes of Health, a federally funded agency, has opened an office called the National Center for Complementary and Alternative Medicine (NCCAM), which currently has a $100 million budget.[6]

But years ago I didn't know I was part of a national healthcare explosion; I only knew I longed for a perspective on cancer that went beyond a nearly total emphasis on removing or destroying malignant cells in my body. I longed for a perspective that would not only give me hope that I could recover my health but would address the *causes* of the physiological breakdown in the first place. As a psychologist, I have been trained to look for causes—to try to understand the forces that shape human behavior while looking for ways to help people function at a higher level. It seemed to me that the answer lay in understanding why my incomparable immune system, with its lymphocytes, macrophages, and natural killer cells, had faltered in doing what it does naturally—protecting my body from infection and dread disease. What had caused its suppression?

ALL OF US HAVE CANCER CELLS

Even when we are in the best of health, all of us walk around every day with about three hundred cancer cells swimming among the 30 trillion cells in our bodies.[7] The difference between a person "with cancer" and a person with fleeting cancer cells is that in the latter, the immune system eliminates the aberrant cells from the body before they can damage the body or create a tumor. However, as naturopathic physician Joseph Pizzorno explains, "When the immune system is not working well, the result is frequent or chronic infections, chronic fatigue, and eventually, cancer."[8]

I could relate to that. Several years before I discovered I had cancer, I had insomnia, migraines, and profound fatigue. Then three months before I found the lump, I struggled with my first bout of pneumonia, feeling sicker than ever before in my life. When I finally went to the local family doctor, he said something that stopped me in my tracks: "Pneumonia is the disease of run-down, burned-out people." Run-down, burned-out—hey, that described me. Not only was I pushing myself too hard, but I was working with a lot of depressed patients who drained me emotionally. I had just signed a three-book contract with short deadlines, which out of hubris I had convinced myself I could meet. And I was battling the upkeep on a rambling old farmhouse, struggling with a sick mother, and attempting to deal with my husband's unexpected retirement. Add to the mix that I ate the sad, bad American diet and seldom exercised, and I was a sitting duck for chronic disease.

Cancer Says Our Lives Are Out of Balance

Cancer forced me to see that my life was woefully out of balance, and this was suppressing my immune system. As I interviewed others who have struggled with cancer, most told me that prior to the discovery of cancer their lives also were characterized by some degree of chronic stress, often caused by workaholism or a difficult work situation or troubled family relationships. Some of them struggled with marital betrayal or divorce or unresolved childhood wounds. Not a few needed to make peace with the past. Most confessed they took poor care of themselves in the years preceding cancer, neglecting exercise, healthy nutrition, even rest. *Their lives were definitely out of balance.*

What about you? If you have been diagnosed with cancer, can you honestly say you have the work-family issue in balance? Or are you stretched to the max so that you feel you have no time for exercise, a healthy diet, or eight hours of sleep each night? Are you involved in painful, difficult relationships that make you feel powerless at times? Is self-nurture a concept you don't even understand?

According to Michio Kushi, the acknowledged leader of the American macrobiotic community and natural foods movement, "Cancer is not the result of some alien factor over which we have no control. Rather it is simply the product of our own daily behavior, including our thinking, lifestyle, and daily way of eating."[9] Kushi goes on to say that "cancer is only the terminal stage of a long process" of failing to live in harmony with our bodies' needs and with our environment. It is the body's attempt to isolate toxins accumulated over a period of years from our diet and from our environment.

And what about modern medicine's emphasis on removing and eradicating cancer cells? According to Kushi, "We must go beyond looking at cancer at the cellular level and realize that our cells are constantly changing in quality, being nourished and rejuvenated as a result of nourishment and energy coming into them."[10] He adds, "The cell is only the terminal of a long organic process and cannot be isolated from its surroundings and other body functions. Instead of focusing on the cell, we need to change the blood, lymph, and environmental conditions that have created malignant cells."[11]

As I read, I realized that cancer is more than a wake-up call; it is the body's last plaintive cry for help. The tumor is saying, "Change or die."

CANCER SAYS CHANGE AND FIGHT FOR YOUR LIFE

I must admit that when I began to confront the truth of Kushi's words, my initial response was fear and confusion, but I appreciated his emphasis on the individual's responsibility in the whole disease process. Too often the perspective I encountered in the medical community was that cancer was the result of genetics, the environment, or the aging process. The first doctors I worked with didn't want me to believe I had anything to do with the breakdown of my health because then I would feel guilty, as if guilt were the worst of human emotions. Try powerlessness…or hopelessness…or despair. Since I have never felt guilty about getting sick, to be told I had nothing to do with my illness made me feel as if I were a powerless onlooker at a massive train wreck. Unfortunately, the wrecked train was my body.

The truth is, if we have cancer and we believe that the way we live or the way we handle stress or our negative emotions may have suppressed our immune system, then we can make life-enhancing changes. How empowering to believe we can *do* something to help our bodies reclaim health! We can change our diets, omitting junk food and devitalized fruits and vegetables laced with pesticides. We can restructure our whole lives if we desire: reducing or managing stress, examining our toxic relationships, deepening our faith in a God who loves us. Conversely, how devastating to be treated as passive recipients of cancer or as victims of impersonal fate who can do little but follow the advice of experts, submit to their various treatments, and wait to see if the disease recurs.

I don't know about you, but passively waiting to see if cancer would recur was not part of my repertoire. If my diet, lack of exercise, and stressed-out life contributed to the onset of cancer, then I wanted to change my life and give my body its best chance to heal. I could make new choices. After all, when clients sought my help for anxiety and depression, I didn't say to them, "Relax, there's nothing you can do to improve your life. Suffer. Stay in your place of pain and despair." Instead, I tried to empower them, because they were already feeling helpless and hopeless. Invariably I asked, "Are your choices helping or hurting you?" They usually replied that their current choices were hurting them. So we worked together to enable them to make better choices. As my clients made new, healthier choices, they became more assertive and less depressed. Why then couldn't I make new and better choices to attempt to reclaim my health?

Why can't you?

As we begin to make new and better choices, we come to understand that illness—whether it is mental or physical—is a dark messenger sent to tell us that our lives aren't working, that the disease in our bodies is related to the dis-ease in our souls. The psychiatrist M. Scott Peck addresses the concept of illness in his bestseller *The Road Less Traveled*:

> The symptoms and the illness are not the same thing. The illness exists long before the symptoms. Rather than being the illness, the symptoms are the beginning of its cure. The fact that they are unwanted makes them all the more a phenomenon of grace—a gift of God, a message from the unconscious, if you will, to initiate self-examination and repair.[12]

Although Peck is addressing mental illness, his comments also apply to physical illness. The dis-ease in our lives and souls has existed long before the manifestation of cancer's symptom—the tumor. Finding or recognizing the symptom, although terrifying, can put us on the road to recovery. To get well we must refuse to continue living lives that are out of touch with our legitimate physical, spiritual, and emotional needs. To fight for our lives we must do what we may be terrified of doing: change.

We must change our thoughts. Our attitudes toward others and ourselves. Our habits. Our relationships. Our diets. We must be willing to radically alter our lives, if necessary, to get well. And we must strengthen our faith in a God who deeply cares about our welfare. I have found in talking to other cancer survivors that many were living lives of "quiet desperation" at the time of their diagnosis. To survive, they recognized they had to make significant changes in their inner and outer lives, and they were willing to do so. In the face of such a formidable foe as cancer, I was not only willing to change, I was eager to work at "self-examination and repair."

Cancer Says Tap into the Healing Power of Faith

While reflection and the necessity of change were easy for me to embrace, Peck's comment that symptoms are a phenomenon of grace was harder for me to accept. Caught up in the horror of cancer, I couldn't see that something so painful, so life threatening could be a gift of grace. Yet it is not unusual for people of faith to view illness as an opportunity to deepen their devotion and grow closer to God. One of my friends says that in her Catholic faith, suffering and sickness are viewed as "the kiss of the cross," a way of communing with Christ and his sufferings. In the seventeenth century, Brother Lawrence, famous for his thin little book of collected letters *The Practice of the Presence of God,* certainly believed that sickness bore God's imprimatur. Brother Lawrence said that while the world views sickness as an affliction, he felt sickness was a "gift from God" and "a consequence of his mercy," as well as the means he often employed for our salvation. The friar, who joyfully practiced the presence of God while washing pots and pans in the monastery kitchen, also believed that God is our primary physician and that he wishes to cure us himself.[13]

Although I was a Christian when I discovered I had breast cancer, I confess that at the time I didn't feel loved by God. Not deeply, truly loved. While I went through the motions of reading my Bible and attending church regularly, it seemed God kept his distance and wasn't particularly concerned about my life. At earlier times in my life God had been close and intimate, but the fire had long since gone out of my spiritual life. I had become a driven woman whose thirst for achievement sprang from childhood wounds that left me grasping for an enduring sense of personal worth. And like many who struggle with cancer, I had yet to feel worthy of love, even God's love, just because I existed.

A significant turn in my thinking came after a conversation with my favorite Georgetown professor, Father Daniel O'Connell. Father O'Connell is a linguistic psychologist, a Jesuit priest, and the former chairman of the psychology department at Georgetown. This warm and optimistic man told me he had always lived in freshman dorms so he could be accessible to students who sought him out for late-night conversations. That this accomplished professor and priest regards some of his students as family is obvious. The walls of his office are decorated with dozens of pictures of former students who have invited him to perform their weddings and baptize their babies.

Father O'Connell and I developed a friendship during my seven years as a graduate student. As one of the oldest among my peers, I sought him out as a wise, empathic spiritual advisor who emanated the love of God. But when I asked him for career advice shortly after I was diagnosed, Father Dan replied, "Ah, Brenda. Your life has been about *doing*. Let it be about *being*. Why not let God cherish you?"

Let God cherish me? Had I ever felt cherished by God? Yes, but that was long ago.

And how to focus on *being* rather than *doing* when I lived near Washington, D.C., a city where most people are seeking either power or proximity to power? Where they live harried, frenetic lives? Invariably, whenever I met anyone in that city, he or she asked, "What are you doing?" No one ever asked about my sense of being or the state of my soul. So how was I to get off the fast train and concentrate on being?

Amazingly, this has happened. Deciding to change our lives postcancer, Don and I moved to the Blue Ridge Mountains, trading bumper-to-bumper traffic and high-stress living for whitewater rafting, rambles in the country, and time to focus on being. Today as I work at my computer, I look outside my window and see mountains bathed in sunshine. A hummingbird hovers at the bird feeder. My husband and I have already spent time, separately and together, reading the Bible and praying. Then we took off for our daily quota of sunshine on an early morning hike. As we walked, we looked up into a cloudless, Carolina-blue sky.

In my new life, nature beckons daily. Yesterday I sloshed around in the winter mud on a friend's farm as she and I chased a young pig that had escaped its pen.

We laughed uproariously as we slid into the pen behind the terrified creature. In contrast, my friend Sue called today from Washington, D.C., saying she was clad in her power suit on her way to have lunch with a friend who works at the White House. Stressed, Sue has to fire several employees as her company downsizes. When I told her about yesterday's experience, she wailed, "I need a pig in my life!" I laughed and agreed. Everyone could do with raspberry picking, weekly rambles in the country, and even a pig in his life.

As I have sought healing for my body and soul—and an immersion in nature has been part of that healing experience—I am aware that God has ever been behind the scenes, orchestrating the positive changes in my life, guiding me each step of the way. Early on I found a verse in Psalm 118 that expresses what I hope will be true in my life. These simple words are now seared on my brain and written in my heart: "I will not die but live, and will proclaim what the LORD has done" (verse 17).

As I have discovered, cancer can nudge us to deepen our faith in an intimate, personal God. And when this happens, faith begins its healing alchemy. As abundant research shows, belief in a God who cares about our well-being is powerful medicine for our bodies, souls, and emotions. For those of us who have a vibrant faith in a loving Creator, this is good news, and for those of us who struggle to believe that God knows our name, phone number, and address, cancer gives us an opportunity to draw closer to the Father of all comfort as we walk through the very real valley of the shadow of death.

Then our illness can become a "phenomenon of grace."

CANCER SAYS HEAL YOUR MIND AND EMOTIONS

As part of our cancer journey, we need to make peace with our past. We must rid ourselves of toxic emotions—grudges, resentments, bitterness—so we will not be vulnerable to depression and anxiety, those powerful immunosuppressors. We must eventually forgive those who have hurt us and seek forgiveness if we have wronged others. And we must finally confront any childhood wounds and seek inner healing. Trauma does not just dissipate over time; rather it is locked in some far corner of our primitive brains, outside our conscious awareness but powerful nonetheless. When I interviewed Dr. Mitchell Gaynor, he told me we hold trauma in our bodies and that this is related to cancer.[14] To enhance our ability to heal, then, we must confront any trauma in our past.

Although you may not choose to go into therapy to work through your past, I did. When it came time to confront and exorcise the demons in my past, I worked with a therapist you will meet in a later chapter, Dorothy (Didi) Firman, the director of the Synthesis Center in Amherst, Massachusetts. Shortly after we met, she told me, "You have lived in your head all of your life, but cancer lives in the body." She added that healing of the childhood wounds I sought would come only by working through the past at the experiential, emotional level. After only four hours of working together, I walked out of Didi's office a different woman. I was, after long years of struggle, finally at peace with my emotionally unstable mother. I was at peace with myself.

CANCER SAYS REDISCOVER YOUR
LIFE'S MEANING AND PURPOSE

After decades of working with cancer patients, clinical psychologist Dr. Lawrence LeShan found that years before their tumors were discovered, many experienced a loss of meaning and purpose in their lives. In *Cancer As a Turning Point,* LeShan writes: "In a large majority of the people I saw (certainly not all), there had been, previous to the first noted signs of the cancer, a loss of hope in ever achieving a way of life that would give real and deep satisfaction, that would provide a solid raison d'être, the kind of meaning that makes us glad to get out of bed in the morning and glad to go to bed at night—the kind of life that makes us look forward zestfully to each day and to the future."[15]

How well I remember that feeling. I told myself that the zestful forties had simply been replaced by the mellow fifties, but that wasn't the whole truth. During the years I was pursuing my doctorate at Georgetown, I worked with two presidential commissions and gave speeches on Capitol Hill. I often traveled to New York, Chicago, or Los Angeles to appear on national television shows such as *Larry King Live,* CBS's *This Morning,* and the *Today* show in support of mothers doing their own mothering. I felt keenly that part of my purpose in life was to be an advocate for babies in a culture that devalued both them and their mothers. I united with other impassioned mothers and attempted to change attitudes toward mothering. I had a cause, a worthy cause since I truly believe that babies are at risk for emotional insecurity if they enter day care in that vulnerable first year of life.

Unfortunately, the political climate changed in Washington, D.C., during the early nineties. Suddenly the dynamics of the day-care issue changed. Any public debate about the topic of mother care versus other care either ceased or went underground. I looked for a job in public policy but found nothing that excited me. Also, a nonprofit advocacy group for mothers that I had cofounded and poured my energies into faltered and died.

I turned to psychotherapy as a profession, but the advocate in me struggled as I submerged my personality so that my patients could discover theirs. While my superiors commended me on my work, and many of my patients did well, I longed to resume an advocacy role. In the words of Dr. LeShan, "I could no longer sing my song." I felt I had lost my calling. Once full of zest and excitement, I now had quiet days. Oh, I had moments of happiness, but I was not operating on all cylinders—fully alive.

My life was quietly imploding. I was ripe for cancer.

About a year after I started working with Dr. Shamim, I read about the work of Dr. Keith Block, an integrative oncologist who is the founder and director of the Block Center for Integrative Cancer Care in Evanston, Illinois. Block is the editor in chief of the peer-reviewed medical journal *Integrative Cancer Therapies* and is among the leading experts on integrative cancer care in America. Intrigued by what I read, I traveled to Evanston to see Dr. Block and have him evaluate how I was doing. (By this time you know I love second and third opinions!) When I arrived at the Center, Block's staff told me he had red-eyed it home from Alaska the night before; he had been surfing fifteen- to twenty-foot waves off the coast of Alaska. Although I was apprehensive—yet another oncologist!—Block quickly put me at ease. Since I had already been seen by another internist on his staff and a registered dietitian, we were able to have a focused conversation that proved enlightening and greatly encouraging. He felt I was on a good course with diet and supplements, though he urged further individualized tailoring based on specific biochemical lab testing, and we discussed the pros and cons of tamoxifen as well.

Finally he told me he didn't feel I was in a desperate situation and that with my involvement in my own recovery and continued clinical monitoring, I would probably do well. "But work is too important to you," he said. "You need to find something fun or even thrilling to do." Observing that I was obsessing about the possibility of a recurrence, he continued, "You need to work on being less fearful and reengage in living."

Block then provided me with a comprehensive and strategic integrative plan designed especially for me to improve my odds of avoiding a cancer recurrence. We discussed specific integrative options to consider should I have a future problem. Though he provides low-dose chemotherapy based on circadian timing to reduce toxicity and improve outcome, he did not advise this for my situation. He did advise a personalized nutrition, physical care, and mind-spirit treatment plan. By discussing a long-term road map and providing a comprehensive, integrated medical plan, Block reduced my stress and helped me regain a sense of control over my health and life.

When I left Block's office that day, I felt peaceful. Here was a physician who had documented success in treating cancer patients, even those with recurrent breast cancer. The depth of his clinical experience was evident in every aspect of my care. Easy to talk to, he had answered my questions, providing further advice on keeping my estrogen levels low in light of my resistance to drugs. When I told him I wanted to continue down my unconventional path, he urged aggressive monitoring, which would allow for a less aggressive treatment approach, while he pressed me to adhere carefully to his program and agreed to work with me long term. Moreover, he treated me with respect, something I had yearned for but hadn't always received from physicians I consulted in the Cancer Zone.

As Don and I boarded the train to go home, I let out an audible sigh of relief—grateful I could add this physician with his program and advice to my select team of knowledgeable and compassionate healers and further improve my cancer fight. What I realized that day was that I had started down the path to rediscover my life's sense of meaning and purpose. I had accepted Block's challenge to move beyond fear to zest and enthusiasm—to concentrate on living instead of on the terrifying possibility of dying.

You Can Make a Difference

Perhaps all of this sounds daunting if you are currently reeling from a cancer diagnosis or recovering from surgery or struggling through chemo and radiation. If so, you may feel weak and downright ill. Understand that working to reclaim your health is a gradual process. It's not possible to attempt to heal your body and your life all at once. But if you want a road map through the uncharted territory that is life after cancer, read on. Or if you want to prevent cancer, this book can also help you, alerting you to changes you need to make in your diet, your attitudes, and your lifestyle to maximize your health.

This chapter has been a preview of the rest of the book, which addresses these areas of our lives that we need to change. Part one discusses the care of your amazing body: the need for a radically nutritious diet, daily exercise, time spent in nature, self-nurturance, and detoxification. I have also included a chapter about the famous Hippocrates Institute, a place of healing where, for over fifty years, people with catastrophic cancers have gone.

Part two deals with the mind-body connection in cancer. In her research Dr. Candace Pert, a professor at Georgetown University, found that our emotions communicate with our cells moment by moment. We pay a heavy physiological price for every negative emotion we repress, for every hopeless thought we allow to control our thinking. The burgeoning field of psychoneuroimmunology (which researches the interaction between the mind, the nervous system, and the cells) advocates that "where the head goes, the body follows." In this book you will discover how to heal your mind, eradicate toxic emotions, and strengthen your will to live. You will also learn how to deal with your toxic relationships by either changing them for the better or gently letting them go.

Part three deals with the spirit. Abundant research shows we live half-lives without faith. This section explores the close connection between prayer and recovery from illness, as well as our need for intimacy with God. We can only experience peace of mind, that powerful elixir, when we feel loved and cared for by a God who cherishes us, who calls us by name. When the mind and spirit are at peace, then the immune system is best able to do its healing work. Proverbs 14:30 says, "A heart at peace gives life to the body."

So where do we begin? When we're scrambling to stay alive, the first and best thing we can do is nourish our bodies. We've heard it a zillion times, and it's true—everything we put into our mouths counts, for good or ill. The good news is that a cornucopia of delicious fruits and vegetables is just waiting to strengthen and rebuild our bodies—one mouthful at a time. As you start to eat better, you will feel stronger. This is something you can safely and immediately do for yourself. When I radically altered my diet, I felt empowered. No longer a passive recipient of care from the medical experts, I was engaged in taking radically good care of myself. And you can do the same.

Let's start the healing process—in the kitchen.

RESTORING

THE BODY

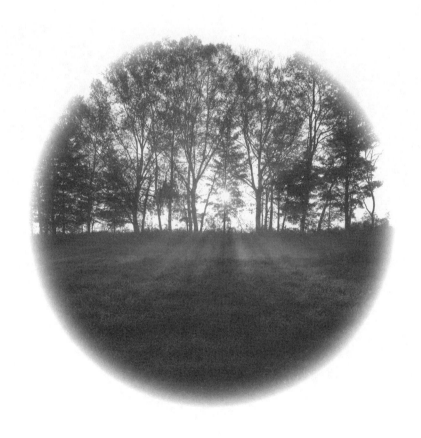

Avoiding the Food Villains

In 1991 six-foot-four Bob Marik, a hard-driving venture capitalist, was going through an extremely stressful period. Not only was he living in Washington, D.C., separated from his family, who had remained in Princeton, New Jersey, but his job was spiraling out of control. "I was working on financial transactions and had been for a protracted time. I would go full throttle all day and deep into the evening, especially when things were not going well."

Bob was aware that the stress was taking a toll on his body and his diet. He started each twelve- to fourteen-hour workday with a bagel, cream cheese, and a pot of coffee. At noon he took time from his demanding work on mergers and acquisitions to ride the elevator down to the first floor and walk outside, where he purchased his usual lunch—a hot dog with ketchup and mustard. At the end of the day, after he had dropped off a package at the nearby FedEx station, Bob would often drive to a local restaurant, where he would order either pasta or a meat entrée. What about fruits and vegetables? Bob told me he ate one or two at the most on any given day. He added, "During that particularly stressful period, I ate just to keep going, and there were lots of days when I ate *no* fruits and vegetables." When he was thirsty, Bob generally consumed one liquid only: the ever-present cup of coffee on his desk. Water? His body hardly knew it existed.

Then one day Bob discovered blood in his urine. Immediately he scheduled an appointment with his internist, who later referred him to a urologist. The diagnosis? Bladder cancer. Initially Bob wasn't particularly troubled about the diagnosis, optimistic thinker that he is, but he became more concerned when he learned that the tumor was embedded in the bladder wall. *That* got his attention. Seeking a second opinion, Bob and his wife, Joan, took the train to New York to the mall-like bastion of cancer treatment, Memorial Sloan-Kettering Cancer Center, where Bob received sobering news. "You have a 25 percent chance of survival," said the oncologist he saw that day. "If you take chemotherapy, your chances increase to 33 percent."

"I wasn't particularly impressed with the slim advantage chemo afforded me," said Bob. "Basically, I just didn't think the difference between 25 and 33 percent was statistically significant." In the end he opted for surgery only. Fortunately, between his diagnosis and second appointment, Bob began to research the role of nutrition in cancer recovery and started to work with nutritionist and former surgeon Dr. Ahmad Shamim. A year later when Bob had a second surgery at Sloan-Kettering for a tumor in his lung—not unusual for metastasized bladder cancer—he had only one rather than the expected hundreds of tumors. Moreover, the tumor was hollow, indicating that it was dying. "That made me feel I was on a good track with the nutrition," said Bob.

In working with Bob to regain his health, Dr. Shamim advised him to give up caffeine, alcohol, all sources of refined sugar, tobacco, sodas, commercial breads and cereals (unless made from organic grains), meat, fried foods, white flour, white rice, and anything containing hydrogenated oil. Instead, the doctor told him to eat a diet rich in fruits, vegetables, whole grains, and legumes (beans). As for dairy, during the past twelve years of healthy living, Bob has eaten only plain yogurt and occasionally low-fat or soy cheese. He has not eaten any meat or fish since 1991. In addition, this man, for whom coffee had been the beverage of choice, now daily consumes almost a quart of fresh vegetable juice, two quarts of cancer-fighting teas (red clover, pau d'arco, and green tea), and a quart of water. "I feel great," says Bob, who has abundant energy and a contagious zest for life.

When Bob went to Memorial Sloan-Kettering recently for his yearly checkup, his oncologist told him, "Bob, I've discussed your case with my oncology residents. You did everything in your cancer treatment I told you *not* to do, and yet look at you. You're a walking miracle."

Bob laughed and replied, "Miracle? I work hard at this."[1]

Food—A Powerful Ally Against Cancer

Contrary to what his oncologist may believe, Bob has based his cancer recovery on good science. In fact, the scientific evidence is flooding in: Ordinary vegetables, fruits, grains, seeds, and nuts—except peanuts—are not only essential for the prevention of heart disease, obesity, diabetes, arthritis, and a host of other ills, but they are literally gifts from God for the prevention of, and possible recovery from, cancer. At a Duke University conference on complementary and alternative medicine, the speakers agreed that the link between cancer and nutrition, which was once treated as folklore, is now considered good science. Currently more than two hundred studies show a reduction of lung, colon, breast, cervix, esophageal, and oral cancers in individuals who regularly consume a plethora of fruits and vegetables.[2]

According to popular science writer Jean Carper:

> Ever since scientists started probing a cancer-diet connection in the 1970s, the antidote to cancer has been coming up "fruits and vegetables," consistently and relentlessly. It is a striking read-my-lips kind of message. In the words of Dr. Peter Greenwald, director of the Division of Cancer Prevention and Control at the National Cancer Institute: "The more fruits and vegetables people eat, the less likely they are to get cancer, from colon and stomach cancer to breast and even lung cancer. For many cancers, persons with high fruit and vegetable intake have about half the risk of people with low intakes."[3]

Massive evidence supports this claim. In fact, some scientists view fruits and vegetables as "a powerful preventive drug that could substantially wipe out the scourge of cancer, just as cleaning up the water supply eliminated past epidemics, such as cholera."[4] So ordinary fruits and vegetables are powerful medicine, not just to prevent cancer but to help those of us struggling to survive the disease and reclaim our health.

Twenty-five hundred years ago Hippocrates, the father of medicine, said, "Let food be your medicine; let medicine be your food." This famous physician, who wrote the Hippocratic oath that every medical student takes upon graduating from medical school, clearly understood just how powerful food is for the human body, both to maintain health and recover from illness. Before I was diagnosed with breast cancer, I had never heard of Hippocrates' nutritional advice, and perhaps neither have you. Unfortunately, many physicians who subscribe to Hippocrates' injunction to "do no harm" do not share his understanding of the healing power of nutrition.

WHAT YOUR DOCTOR MAY NOT KNOW

Numerous cancer survivors have told me that when they asked their oncologists what they should eat during and after chemo, they got vague or evasive answers. One woman who had just finished her first round of chemotherapy for breast cancer said, "I asked my oncologist if he had any nutritional advice, and he replied that I could eat anything in moderation." Unfortunately, moderation doesn't work if you're drinking sodas and eating Twinkies and fast food on a regular basis.

I heard Dr. Mitchell Gaynor tell an audience of healthcare professionals and cancer patients that when he was in medical school, he signed up for a course on nutrition. The first day of class his professor walked in, and looking out at the eager faces of his students, he held up a taco. "See the taco shell? That's your grain. The beef? That's your protein. The lettuce and tomato? Those are your vegetables. And the sour cream? That's your dairy." With that, the professor tossed the taco into the wastebasket and said, "Now for hard science."[5] Gaynor told this story not only to illustrate why he hadn't learned about nutrition in medical school but also to point out the attitude that professor and others have had toward the "soft science" of nutrition. Until recently, most medical schools have not offered substantive courses in nutrition, which is why most doctors don't have nutritional guidelines to give their patients.

In addition, Dr. Keith Block believes that the heart of the problem is that doctors eat terrible food during their years of training. "When the food available to medical students and residents in American hospitals is of the quality that promotes ill health, one can only wonder if even the best medical education is enough to override what is clearly a topsy-turvy system." He continued, "Conventional approaches have disease care at the foundation and health as an afterthought. What is needed is health and good nutrition at the foundation and then disease care superimposed on top of this solid base. Patients will not only tolerate conventional care better, but every indication says they will have better outcomes."[6]

Block speaks from personal experience. He started investigating the healing power of food twenty-five years ago when, as a medical student, he suffered from chronic migraines and a gastric disorder that got worse with conventional treatment.[7] Desperate, he became his own doctor and turned to holistic therapies and a macrobiotic diet. As he cured his own maladies, he started to explore botanical medicine, acupuncture, and nutrition.

Block, who believes that a low-fat, high-fiber, plant-based diet can either slow or reverse tumor growth, has devised a whole-foods diet for his patients that stresses complex carbohydrates, whole-grain cereals, vegetables, and legumes. In a culture of fad diets that shun carbs, Block believes that complex (not refined) carbs should account for 50 percent of daily caloric intake. Since scientific evidence shows that lowering fat impacts survival rates by starving tumors, Block's patients consume a diet that derives only 10-20 percent of caloric intake from fat of the healthy omega-3 variety, mostly from flax and fish. Block also advocates a high-fiber diet, consisting of whole grains, legumes, and phytochemically rich organic fruits and vegetables, that not only retards the development of tumors but transports carcinogens out of the body posthaste. Protein? Block believes that patients should consume low to moderate amounts of protein daily, adjusted to weight and body composition. For example, a 120-pound, five-feet-seven-inch woman combating breast cancer should consume sixty grams, while that same woman in remission five years later needs fifty grams. Enough to nourish the body without feeding the tumor. Forget the Atkins diet. The average American consumes 120 grams of protein each day, which can damage the liver over the long term.

Does Block's diet really help cancer patients? Block's patients not only feel better eating a plant-based diet, but many are long-term cancer survivors.

Fortunately, a sea change is coming in conventional medicine as more physicians are learning about the power of nutrition in treating cancer. Prestigious teaching hospitals affiliated with major universities like Harvard, Emory, Duke, the University of Michigan, Stanford, and the University of North Carolina are offering nutritional help for their patients as part of their integrative medicine programs, and at conferences and in their publications, physicians are educating their colleagues about the clinical relevance of medicinal herbs and nutrition.

CONFESSIONS OF A CONVERT

Before I discovered I had breast cancer, I thought I ate a pretty decent diet. In college I had worked for an early health-food devotee, Marty Clansky. Marty, deeply influenced by the nutritional guru of the fifties and sixties, Adele Davis, suggested that I eat whole grains and lots of fruits and veggies for better health. Unfortunately, Davis was also a proponent of high meat consumption because of that magical elixir protein. I was not surprised to learn several years ago that Davis, herself a high meat eater, had died of cancer.

Since I had grown up on a high-fat, high-sugar Southern farm diet with a grandmother who baked two pies each day and plied my grandfather with artery-clogging dishes (Granddaddy, a fighter, succumbed to his third heart attack), the emphasis on whole grains, fruits, and veggies was a vast improvement. When I had my own family, we maintained this diet, along with lots of meat and dairy, until my obstreperous teenagers challenged our no-soda, no-junk-food policy. Weary of holding the nutritional line at home, in grad school I began to reward myself with food I had seldom eaten—Kit-Kats (18 grams of fat), an occasional Big Mac (30 grams of fat), and potato chips (10 grams of fat). After all, the hours were long and the coursework demanding, so I deserved to eat whatever I wanted, right? In addition, I increased my coffee consumption and started to drink a daily soda (loaded with caffeine and 27 grams of sugar) as I headed off for Georgetown University's Lauinger Library for hours of work. Did I gain weight? Surprisingly, no. But I felt lousy much of the time.

When I worked out at the local spa, I jokingly told my friends that I was an eighty-year-old woman trapped in a forty-nine-year-old body. And I meant it. I told myself that I was perimenopausal and therefore estrogen and calcium deprived. So I increased my dairy and meat consumption (looking for energy, right?), and thus began a vicious cycle. The more dairy and meat I ate, the worse I felt. The worse I felt, the more dairy and meat I consumed. *It never occurred to me that my lifestyle, and particularly my diet, had anything to do with how I felt.* So while I was earning As in my psychology courses, I was garnering Fs in the care and feeding of my own body.

No longer. Once I stopped eating food that hurt my body and made every morsel I ate part of a plant-based diet, which I named my Staying-Alive Diet, I began to feel better and recover my health. Today I feel great. At sixty-two, I have the energy level I had twenty-five years ago. After being an insomniac for fifteen years, I have rediscovered immune-enhancing sleep. My blood pressure has dropped from 145/95 to 110/72. I have lost the twenty pounds I gained on hormone replacement therapy. (I stopped taking HRT when I learned I had cancer.) My total cholesterol, which had hovered at 235, is now 180.

I not only feel better, I look better. My once lifeless and lusterless hair has body and sheen—something my hair colorist couldn't give it no matter how hard she tried. My nails, which used to be fragile and pale, are strong and pink, as healthy, normal nails should be. My skin? I moisturize from within with eight glasses of *pure* water daily, along with cups of decaffeinated green tea and more than a quart of vegetable juice made with my Champion juicer.

When I had a facial recently at the new Grove Park Inn Spa—a gift from my younger daughter—the thirty-five-year-old aesthetician told me my skin was firm and healthy looking, uncommon for someone my age. I told her my largely vegetarian diet and conscientious juicing were responsible. As I prepared to leave, she asked, "What was the name of that juicer?" I felt enormously flattered.

What has caused this positive transformation? Using the guidelines from my nutritionist, Dr. Shamim, and Dr. Keith Block, along with my review of the scientific evidence, I radically purged my kitchen of all the bad foods and fake foods that were destroying my body, and then I began purchasing only those foods that research showed would have an anticancer effect, supporting my immune system and restoring my health. I dared to believe I could defy my oncologist's grim statistics, reverse the process of disease in my body, and regain my health.

Say Farewell to Food Villains

To get well or stay well we must eliminate the food villains—salt, white sugar, white flour, white rice, fried foods, bad fats, colas—from our diet. In addition, we must refuse to eat processed foods that contain precarcinogenic hydrogenated oils and are utterly devoid of nutritional value. Feeling virtuous about eating low-fat, low-sugar snacks? Don't. With their trans fatty acids and chemical sweeteners, these foods are some of the worst offenders. That includes most, if not all, of our snack foods. But we can't stop there. We must also eliminate all caffeine, dairy, meat, shellfish, and other destroyers of our health, such as those sugar substitutes like aspartame (NutraSweet), which Dr. Shamim says can "cause brain and eye damage."[8] And if you're basically healthy? Then commit to removing most of these foods from your diet.

Stunned? Let's look at each of these villains to understand why avoiding them is critical to our health.

Salt

Americans are addicted to heavily salted foods, so much so that those of us who succumb to cancer have altered the sodium-potassium ratio in our cells. While the healthy cell has a sodium-potassium ratio of 1:4, the cancer cell is an unhealthy 4:1. By overconsuming salt (and all processed foods are loaded with it), we have, according to nutritionist Dr. Patrick Quillin, literally changed "the battery of life."[9] Quillin suggests that every cell in our bodies has an electrical charge that is generated by the concentration of potassium on the inside of the cell and the sodium chloride on the outside. The electrical potential that is created allows both oxygen and nutrients to enter the cell while toxins flow out. When we consume too much salt, changes occur in the electrolyte balance, and "the cell begins to 'secede from the union' and develop its own 'country' of fermenting anaerobic rapidly growing cancer cells."[10]

This means that if you have an active cancer, you have cancer cells literally swimming in a salty soup. So what you want to do is reverse the sodium-potassium ratio by eradicating salt from your diet, especially in the early months after diagnosis, and literally flooding your cells with potassium. If you don't believe you use much salt, read the label of everything that comes from a box or can. You'll be surprised at how much hidden salt you consume throughout the day.

The late Dr. Max Gerson, whose Gerson Therapy has been followed by cancer patients worldwide—often with amazing results—believed that cancer patients desperately need to follow a saltless diet. He said that this allows salt to be excreted from the body while the patient increases his consumption of potassium, the mineral antagonist to salt. Recent studies of the Gerson Therapy have found that a salt-free diet with high potassium intake may help damaged cells return to their precancerous condition.[11]* In essence, research shows that you can turn "on and off metastasis by altering the sodium to potassium ratio" in your diet.[12]

And where do you find potassium? In fruits and veggies. A world of high potassium vegetables exists—from watercress to Swiss chard—that can help your struggling cells.

Sugar

According to Rex Russell, M.D., in *What the Bible Says About Healthy Living,* the average American consumes 150 pounds of refined sugar yearly. Some sugarholics go so far as to pack away a pound per day, or 350 pounds a year.[13] American foodstuffs literally abound with sugar, including beverages, bottled juices, canned fruits, pastries, doughnuts, ice cream, ketchup, boxed cereals, and fast foods.

Yet refined sugar is one of the most dangerous things an individual with cancer can consume because *cancer feeds on sugar.* In fact, Dr. Patrick Quillin states that when you have cancer, consuming sugar is like "throwing gasoline on a smoldering fire."[14] Why is this so? Sugar raises blood glucose levels, and blood glucose feeds cancer cells. In your fight against cancer, it is imperative to avoid sugar and to use even natural sweeteners like rice syrup and barley malt sparingly. *Sparingly.* In the beginning I occasionally used barley malt as a sweetener since the body metabolizes it at a slower pace and it is less disruptive to blood glucose levels. But I left other

---

* All references attributed in the endnotes to this source are from *The Gerson Therapy.* Copyright © 2001 by Dr. Morton Walker and The Gerson Institute. Published by arrangement with Kensington Publishing Corp. All rights reserved. Reprinted by permission of Citadel Press / Kensington Publishing Corp. www.kensingtonbooks.com.

sweeteners alone for a long time. I try to avoid eating anything that has white sugar. Recently, when I attended the Hippocrates Health Institute, the number one cancer health spa in the world, I learned that the codirectors do not advocate even eating fruit in the early stages after the diagnosis, and the only sweetener they recommend is the herb stevia, which does not affect blood sugar.

Additionally, sustained high sugar intake suppresses the immune system.[15] I remember the day I learned that the sugar in a single soda (twenty-seven grams) could suppress my immune system for *four* hours. For several years I had been a one-a-day soda consumer, but no longer. I have given up sodas forever.

Of course, even if you stop using white sugar, it (like salt) is hidden in all processed food. That's why it's important to eat fresh, unprocessed food. Just remember when you read the sugar content of a processed item that four grams of sugar equal one teaspoon. Once you start reading the labels, you may be appalled, as I was, at how much sugar is in the boxes and cans of food in the grocery store. But the food industry in this country is clever. It knows that we're addicted to salt and sugar, and it panders to that addiction.

White Flour

White flour has no fiber and absolutely no nutritional value. It is nothing but empty calories. All the goodness of wheat—the germ, the bran—has been removed through processing, so each time you eat *anything* made with white flour, you are robbing your body of important nutrients. That means that bagels, breads, muffins, doughnuts, cakes, pies, pasta, pancakes—if made from any form of white flour—undermine your health and do not aid your battle against cancer. White flour also lacks fiber, which is part of the reason approximately 70 percent of Americans struggle with constipation. Finally, because white flour products have no nutritional value, they fail to shut down the mechanism in our brain that controls satiety. That's why some people can eat slice after slice of white bread and increase their girth without ever feeling satisfied. When you choose to eat bread, make sure it is made with whole wheat, rye, kamut, millet, or spelt flour with no preservatives or emulsifiers. As one nutritionist said, "The bread should be so dense that it thumps when you drop it on the counter."

If you are allergic to wheat, you may want to switch to bread made from kamut or spelt flour. Spelt is an ancient grain and highly nutritious. I love spelt products and rarely eat whole wheat because of its allergy-producing potential.

Dairy

We need our daily quota of milk, right? At least that's what the dairy industry would have us believe with their celebrity-studded "Got Milk?" commercials. Wrong. According to Harvey and Marilyn Diamond, authors of *Fit for Life,* "Milk is the most political food in America."[16] Billions are spent yearly in support of the dairy industry. The Diamonds state that cows don't drink cow's milk, nor should we. That's right. Only calves consume cow's milk and then only until they are weaned. But we consume milk and its products throughout our lives even though the enzymes rennin and lactase, which are essential to digesting milk, disappear from our bodies after age three! So what happens when adults drink milk? The casein in the milk coagulates in the stomach and forms hard-to-digest curds that put a huge burden on the body. As adults we simply can't digest milk, and undigested food wreaks havoc in our bodies.

Additionally, dairy consumption encourages the formation of mucus in the system, and this mucus coats the mucus membranes.[17] Why is this bad? According to Harvey and Marilyn Diamond, mucus is a highly acidic byproduct of milk digestion that is stored in the body, squandering our vital energy.[18] They write: "They next time you are going to dust your home, smear some paste all over everything and see how easy it is to dust."[19] That's what mucus does inside our bodies. Every time I hear someone with a guttural voice or see a baby with mucus coming out of her nose (and her mother says she doesn't have a cold), I think *dairy.* We don't need to overload our bodies with mucus when we're fighting cancer; we want to maximize our system's ability to fight cancer cells and infections.

In addition, Dr. Keith Block states that "milk carries the diseases, viruses (bovine C type), and bacteria of the host animal." To counter this, the dairy industry feeds cows antibiotics as well as the drug sulfamethazine, which may cause cancer. Also, Block notes that dietary fat, particularly dairy fat, greatly increases the risk of breast cancer.[20] One Japanese study found that commercial milk that had been pasteurized and homogenized actually enhanced the development of breast tumors.[21]

In an interview Block told me that milk products contain saturated fats and casein—both of which have cancer-promoting effects. "Dairy also contains omega-6 fatty acids, promoting the wrong environment to fight a malignancy. Fighting cancer requires an optimally functioning immune system. Dairy products place an added burden on a patient's already compromised immune system."[22]

In addition to being an immune burden, milk contains contaminants, such as DES (diethylstilbestrol), which is used to promote rapid growth in cattle, and it also contains pesticides, industrial contaminants, and heavy metals.[23] The bottom line? Milk is not something you want to put in your body whether you have cancer or not.

What about milk's vaunted contribution of calcium to the body? Harvey and Marilyn say that the calcium in cow's milk is much coarser than in human milk and is tied up with casein, which prevents the calcium from being absorbed. Then where do we get our calcium? All those delicious green leafy vegetables and raw nuts, as well as raw sesame seeds and kelp, contain calcium.[24]

So what do you put on your oatmeal or other whole-grain cereal? You can use almond milk or soy milk or rice milk as alternatives. I use a product called Rice Dream, a brown rice derivative, and haven't had a glass of cow's milk in nearly six years. This change in my diet has brought other benefits as well. When I stopped consuming dairy, my digestive problems—the bloating and roiling—disappeared. Also, the mucus that gave me a gravelly voice and required me frequently to clear my throat vanished. I feel worlds better than when I was a cheeseaholic and milk consumer.

But what may be even worse news for some people is that Dr. Shamim believes ice cream is a "harmful nonfood" that should not be eaten by adults or given to children. Sigh. But you can find nondairy alternatives in the freezer section of your organic market.

Meat

Now I know that the subject of meat consumption hits close to the jugular for most Americans. We love our beef or, if we're purists, our chicken. And consuming fast food is a national pastime. When the lovable founder of Wendy's, Dave Thomas, died of liver cancer at sixty-nine, we honored his memory by flooding into Wendy's restaurants nationwide. As I read about Thomas's sad and untimely death, I noted that his favorite Wendy's meal was a "single with cheese, mustard, pickle, onion; fries; chili; Frosty; Diet Coke."[25]

Unfortunately, fast foods are inordinately high in fat and sodium while low in calcium and fiber. Although they may taste good and are conveniently located on nearly every block in America, they ultimately damage our bodies. They not only lack nutrition but are high in protein, with some of them providing 50 to 100 percent of the RDA (recommended daily allowance) for protein consumption. Yet research shows that high consumption of protein is related to cancer, osteoporosis, and heart disease.[26]

I can understand if you're skeptical or less than enthusiastic about giving up meat. When one of my daughters came home from college declaring herself a vegetarian, I rolled my eyes and thought, *Oh brother! We paid good money for this?* Yet when I was diagnosed with breast cancer, independently both Dr. Shamim and Dr. Block told me to stop eating *all* meat immediately and to abstain from meat consumption indefinitely.

Why is meat such a problem? For one thing, unless it's organic, beef is loaded with antibiotics and hormones, particularly estrogens, that make cows grow faster and plumper. And those hormones and antibiotics don't just disappear once the cow is slaughtered. Also, red meat has been linked to colon cancer and prostate cancer. One large medical study of colorectal and breast cancer in twenty-four European countries found that cancer rates rose with the consumption of animal fat.[27] A seventeen-year study in Japan found that heavy meat eaters were more vulnerable to cancers of the pancreas, colon, lung, and breast. Also, eating fried, grilled, smoked, or cured meat may greatly boost your chances of getting pancreatic cancer.

Dr. Dean Ornish, who advocates a vegan diet (no animal foods, fish, or dairy) for his heart and prostate cancer patients, says this about meat consumption:

> When you eat a lot of meat, it takes a long time for it to make its way
> through your digestive tract. As it putrefies and decays, your breath smells
> bad, your sweat smells bad, and your bowels smell bad. Not very attractive.[28]

In addition, in *Eat More, Weigh Less,* Dr. Ornish says that meat is high in cholesterol and clogs the arteries. It's also high in saturated fat, which raises your blood cholesterol, and it's low in antioxidants. He states further that "nonvegetarian women have 50 percent higher blood estrogen levels than vegetarians do."[29] This is bad news, particularly since high levels of estrogen are linked to breast tumors.[30]

Got the picture? Believe me, if you're fighting for your life, eating meat isn't worth the risk. And if you want to prevent cancer? Then rethink your diet and ask why you're eating meat since it isn't essential for health. You steak lovers may be shaking your heads in disbelief, but I promise you that if you stop eating meat for several weeks, you will experience increased energy, a sense of well-being, and freedom from bloating—all of which should convince you to move toward a plant-based diet. Then when someone asks, "Where's the beef?" you can respond, "Who cares?"

And if you think you can just substitute chicken for hormonized red meat, think again. An article in the *New York Times* titled "What If Cipro Stopped Working?" stated that Bayer makes an antibiotic called Baytril, which is used worldwide in chicken production.[31] It is added to the chickens' drinking water during the last weeks before slaughter whether they are healthy or not.

Why does this create a danger for humans? When we eat meat laced with antibiotics, our bodies create drug-resistant bacteria so that if we need an antibiotic in an emergency, it may not be effective.[32] For example, Baytril interferes with the effectiveness of Cipro, an antibiotic used in treating anthrax post-September 11. Because antibiotics destroy the good bacteria in the gut and create an overgrowth of candida or yeast, which depresses our immune system, we must be careful about overconsuming antibiotics. So widespread is the use of antibiotics in our agricultural animals that the Union of Concerned Scientists has said that as many as 70 percent of all the antibiotics produced in America are fed to healthy livestock for growth production.[33] Even McDonald's is phasing out the routine use of antibiotics to promote animal growth. The company has asked all its suppliers, by the end of 2004, to use antibiotics only to heal sick livestock. The company motivation? "To protect public health."[34] While this certainly is a move in the right direction, the best way we can control our overconsumption of antibiotics is to move from a meat-based diet to, yes, you guessed it, a plant-based diet.

Fat

Because I learned soon after my cancer diagnosis that research has found that breast cancer is linked to a high-fat diet, I became wary of all fats, a tough place to be for a former fats lover and high-meat consumer. Then Dr. Shamim explained, "Ah, but there are good fats and bad fats," and proceeded to educate me about different kinds of fat.

I learned, for instance, that the food we eat has a mixture of omega-6 fatty acids and omega-3 fatty acids. Omega-6 fatty acids are found in margarine, vegetable oils—like corn oil, safflower oil, and sunflower oil—and processed foods. Virtually all our snack foods are loaded with omega-6 fatty acids. Omega-3 fatty acids, on the other hand, are found in cold-water fish such as salmon, blue fish, mackerel, sardines, and herring, as well as in some plants, like flax, hemp, and soybeans. While we need both omega-6s and omega-3s in our diet, unfortunately most Americans consume far too much of the omega-6 variety, and this promotes diseases. According to science writer Jean Carper, "If your cells are flooded with omega-6 fatty acids, the resulting oversupply of overactive prostaglandins is apt to run amok, generating disease. If you have sufficient omega-3 fatty acids, they can check or cool down the arachidonic engine that is spewing out the disease-producing eicosanoids."[35] That is, the omega-3s, the "stars," counter the negative, disease-producing effects of too many omega-6s.

Because "patients don't have any idea where they stand" in terms of their omega-3 to omega-6 ratio, Block recommends that those struggling with cancer get a set of tests to assess their levels of oxidation, inflammation, immune function, and other areas affecting their condition in order to precisely individualize their clinical program. This set of tests will help your cancer doctor work with you to maintain a better environment, including an optimal ratio of omega-3 to omega-6 fatty acids to support healing rather than malignant growth. Block states, "Getting your fatty acid ratio right is critical, not only to reduce resistance to treatment, but also to improve outcome."

Another kind of fat, one you should eliminate from your diet, is trans fat. Trans fatty acids, which are found in most snack foods, are dangerous for your health. Block told me, "Trans fatty acids are among the most harmful substances one can ingest. Trans fatty acids gum up the enzymes needed for fatty acid metabolism.

This can lead to a host of adverse health effects, including inflammation. This is not only related to cardiac disease but to various cancers as well. Trans fatty acids weaken a healthy cell and make it more vulnerable to disease, and it can take a cancer cell and make it more impenetrable, like a fortress, and thereby allow it to better withstand natural and conventional therapies, much to the patient's disadvantage."

Staying Alive—With Food

So what should you eat to prevent or survive cancer? That should be evident by now. Your new diet should be a primarily plant-based, whole-foods diet rich in complex carbohydrates. These foods include brown rice, whole grains, vegetables, fruit, and beans. (Forget processed food in cans and boxes.) You should also eat as much raw food as you can comfortably digest—fresh fruits and salads loaded with at least seven or eight chopped vegetables. And you should eat as much organic food as possible to limit the pesticide load on your body. What happens when you limit salt, sugar, dairy, and meat in your diet? Amazingly, you cleanse your palate so that simple fruits and vegetables taste wonderful, especially if they are organically grown in good soil. And your body shouts hallelujah. As Dr. Gaynor explains:

> What happens to your body if you eat enough broccoli trees and cabbage bunches, carrots and tomatoes, soy foods, fish oils, onions, apples, garlic, mushrooms, ginseng, ginger, vitamins, minerals, cereal grasses, cups of green tea…? Does your body actually change? I know that it does.
>
> Your body politely says, "Thank you," and begins to live at a far higher level of health and energy than most of the other bodies around you.
>
> Moreover, when treated this way, *your body builds up a formidable capacity to crush cancers.* Crushing cancers is a big part of its proper business.[36]

Although Dr. Gaynor is talking about prevention of cancer, diet can have a powerful effect on those struggling to recover from the disease. In my travels I have met a number of cancer survivors who, like Bob Marik, have utilized diet in their recovery. Tom Beamon, a metalsmith who lives with his wife, Pat, near the top of a high mountain with a gorgeous view of a rich valley in western North Carolina, believes he is alive today because of his faith in God and his adoption of a radically nutritious diet.

One sunny day I drove up the mountain to the spacious log home he and Pat built, a home filled with American-Indian artifacts as well as Tom's art. As we three sipped our green tea and marveled at the view, Tom told me the following story:

> Three years ago this month I was diagnosed with bladder cancer about a week after I noticed I was sitting in my workroom in a pool of blood. When I went to the urologist, he ordered an MRI and later told me that I had bladder cancer, grade 3. The MRI also revealed the presence of four tumors. I went to the pit of hell, and it was the coldest, nastiest place I had ever been. Unfortunately, while the urologist removed most of the cancer, he told me he would need to perform a second surgery in six weeks to get the rest.
>
> What was my diet like the year before I was diagnosed? It was wretched. We had sold our home and were renovating a small house while we built our mountain home at the same time. For six months we ate fast food every night. Also, I was "Mr. Cheese" and drank nearly a quart of milk as well as four to eight cups of coffee each day. I consumed very little water.
>
> But all of this has changed. Prior to learning I had cancer, Pat and I had heard about the Hallelujah Diet, which is basically a raw foods diet. So after my first surgery, we decided to give it a try. Following the Hallelujah Diet meant I drank eight to nine glasses of carrot juice daily, ate fruit until noon, had a nutritious salad for lunch, and then ate a salad and potatoes or rice for dinner. My diet, which consisted of 80 percent raw food and 20 percent cooked food, was definitely vegan.
>
> After six weeks on the Hallelujah Diet, I went in for my second surgery, and I was as clean as a whistle. No residual cancer. My doctor was surprised but not overtly inquisitive, and when I told him about my dietary changes, he replied, "Well, whatever works."

While Tom's story can be labeled anecdotal evidence, as is the case of all the interviews with cancer survivors in this book, the good news is that with only surgery and radical dietary changes he remains cancer free. His story encourages me, and I have included it to encourage you as well.

Food is miracle medicine. When we eliminate all the foods that harm us and concentrate on foods that nourish and heal, our bodies take notice. Not only do we begin to feel much better, but we may increase our odds of surviving cancer.

But let's get practical. I remember being overwhelmed at the prospect of radical dietary changes during the early weeks after my surgery when I still felt lousy. So we want to make these dietary changes as easy as possible. As you eliminate the food villains, you will need a plan to consume the stars in your anticancer diet and make sure you get the five to nine servings of fruits and vegetables that the National Cancer Institute says we all need to consume daily. Remember, that's just their guideline for cancer *prevention*—so how can you work on cancer *survival?* And how can you radically change your diet without losing your appetite and killing your social life?

Keep reading!

THE STAYING-ALIVE DIET

The average age…of a meat eater is 63. I am on the verge of 85 and still work as hard as ever.… I am trying to die, but I simply cannot do it. A single beefsteak would finish me, but I cannot bring myself to swallow it. I am oppressed with a dread of living forever. This is the only disadvantage of vegetarianism.

GEORGE BERNARD SHAW

If I am what I eat, then I am fast, cheap, and easy.
SIGN AT A TOYOTA REPAIR SHOP IN ASHEVILLE, N.C.

Years of patient care have convinced me that a therapeutic nutrition plan tailored to one's illness and clinical needs is essential to recovery.

DR. KEITH BLOCK

Your x-rays show the large grapefruit tumor on your left lung is asbestos cancer or mesothelioma," said Margie Levine's surgeon calmly. "It is a deadly cancer. Unfortunately, we have no cure. We can only palliate. Surgery is brutal and the recovery long and painful. You may want to forgo treatment and live out your remaining months with dignity and quality of life. Only you can make the decision."[1]

When he delivered his diagnosis, the surgeon didn't know that Margie Levine is a fighter. After two exploratory surgeries, one major operation, five inpatient rounds of chemotherapy, and twenty-five radiation sessions, she is today, more than thirteen years later, the "world's longest living survivor of mesothelioma lung cancer."[2] In her book *Surviving Cancer,* Levine writes that she took charge of her own recovery and that one of the most significant things she did to boost her immune system was to eat a radically nutritious diet.

After reviewing medical research, Levine elected to eat the diet that a plethora of studies shows keeps cancer at bay. She says she "overdoses on veggies." Among the vegetables she regularly keeps in her kitchen are carotenoid-rich carrots, yams, squash, pumpkins, and turnips. She also eats leafy greens daily, choosing from romaine lettuce, arugula, collard greens, and kale. Because research shows that broccoli is a powerhouse in fighting cancer, Levine says, "Whereas I read that the average American eats seven pounds of broccoli a year, I eat seven pounds each *week.*"[3] Levine is aware that broccoli, a member of the cruciferous family, is rich in sulforaphane, an enzyme stimulant that helps rid our bodies of carcinogens.

In addition, this woman eats abundant salads that contain garlic, onions, cabbage, and fresh, grated ginger. She maximizes her fruit intake, focusing on seasonal fruits, and keeps bananas and oranges in her home throughout the year.

Levine's dietary approach is working! She's still alive. "Overdosing on veggies" is a scientific approach that not only can help prevent cancer but may help an ailing body recover. During recent years scientists have identified literally thousands of natural compounds with cancer-fighting potential in ordinary foods. Fruits and vegetables, loaded with phytochemicals with cancer-zapping ingredients, antioxidants, vitamins, and minerals, need to become the core of any anticancer diet, as scores of cancer survivors have discovered.

Recently I spoke with Dr. Rex Russell, an invasive radiologist and author of the excellent book *What the Bible Has to Say About Healthy Living.* He told me that twenty-five years ago he was diagnosed with melanoma. But about six months prior to his diagnosis, he had started a new dietary approach, stressing fruits, vegetables, and grains. In addition, he took one gram of vitamin C each day. When he got the pathology report back after surgery, he read, "It is very unlikely that the patient will have a recurrence of this disease since six layers of healthy cells were surrounding the lymphatic cells, fighting the cancer." When I asked him how he interpreted the pathologist's comments, Dr. Russell said he felt that his healthy diet had protected him.[4] Fruits, grains, and veggies to the rescue!

EAT ACROSS THE "RAINBOW"

When I began to commit to an anticancer diet, I decided to eat those dark, richly colored vegetables that my research indicated packed the most cancer-fighting potential. I learned that I needed to eat not only a variety of vegetables daily but in a greater quantity than I had ever consumed in my life.

To be sure I get the quantity I need—the five to nine fresh fruits and veggies every day—I drink at least a quart of fresh vegetable juice each day. Every day I fill my Champion juicer with carrots, parsley, celery, and a small beet and start juicing. Delicious! In addition, I eat one or two salads daily with five to seven chopped vegetables plus spinach and different lettuces (no iceberg, please, since it has zero nutritional value!). Sometimes I have an all-fruit lunch with a small handful of almonds or walnuts for protein. For dinner I lightly steam an assortment of chopped vegetables, which I eat with brown rice, spelt pasta, tortillas, or a sweet potato.

To be sure I get the needed variety, I try to eat across the "rainbow." What do I mean by that? As you shop the produce aisles, look for deep, rich colors. For *red*, reach for tomatoes, watermelon, red peppers, red apples, beets, red cabbage, radishes, and red grapes. For *orange*, pick up sweet potatoes, carrots, butternut squash, oranges, and tangerines. Look for rich, deep *greens* in Swiss chard, mustard greens, green peppers, spinach, collard greens, asparagus, parsley, cilantro, watercress, peas, green beans, kale, okra, Chinese cabbage, broccoli, green cabbage, Brussels sprouts, green grapes, celery, pears, and all the luscious and varied dark green lettuces. What about *yellow?* Get lemons, bananas, yellow squash, grapefruit, and yellow onions. And don't forget *white:* garlic, cauliflower, parsnips, daikon radishes, and turnips, to name a few.

BUY ORGANIC

As you're choosing which fruits and vegetables to buy, consider buying organic. The pesticide use in this country and around the world is astonishing. *An Alternative Medicine Definitive Guide to Cancer* states that since 1945 pesticide use in America has increased tenfold. Over four hundred pesticides are currently used on our food supply in this country. For example, "In 1995, 1.2 billion pounds were dumped on crop lands, forests, lawns, and fields."[5]

Not only is pesticide use skyrocketing, but the types of pesticides applied to food are expanding: "Worldwide, in the past 50 years, some 15,000 chemical compounds and more than 35,000 different formulations have come into use as pesticides."[6] While the United States has banned many of these pesticides, we sell them to Third-World countries and then import and consume their pesticide-laden fruits and veggies. These countries use DDT with abandon, which is especially harmful. Women who develop breast cancer tend to have a high level of PCBs (pollutants) and DDE, a derivative of DDT, in the fatty tissue of their breasts while women without breast cancer do not.[7] Since the seventies, a number of studies have associated breast cancer with DDT and other pesticides. Ten years after Israel banned DDT and PCBs, breast-cancer deaths in that country dropped sharply, with a 30 percent drop in mortality for women younger than forty-four and an 8 percent decline overall.[8]

Bringing the argument closer to home, in April 2003 a *USA Today* article reported that two studies have found contaminated lettuces containing the chemical perchlorate in a few counties out West that are irrigated by the Colorado River. This touches our lives since 20 percent of the country's lettuce comes from this region for six months a year. Perchlorate not only affects the thyroid gland, but it can also disrupt thyroid production.[9]

The truth is, when you buy conventional fruits and vegetables, you have no idea what you're eating, how much pesticide residue is left on the produce and is inside the produce, and whether it will ultimately hurt you. The best way to protect yourself is to buy organic.

Granted, organic food is more expensive and harder to find, but you may discover that once you have eliminated meat, junk food, snack foods, and fake foods (like butter, sugar, and egg substitutes) from your diet, you'll have more money to spend on organic fruits and vegetables. Look for some of the leading chain stores, such as Whole Foods, Earth Fare, or Wild Oats. And if you don't have a local organic grocery store, check the aisles of your conventional supermarket. Many now stock organic produce and foodstuffs in response to customer demand. If yours doesn't, speak to the store manager to see if he or she would be willing to do so.

And if none of these options work? Research to find the closest organic chain. Even if it's a couple of hours away, your health is well worth the trip. You can consolidate shopping and go once or twice a month.

Look for organic farmers' markets, which run much of the year, or local farmers who sell direct to the public. You may be able to join a local organic food co-op and have produce delivered straight to your door. If that fails, you can grow your own vegetables in a sunny corner of the backyard. You'll want to be certain, however, that your neighbors aren't treating their lawns with chemicals, as this will defeat the purpose of growing your own garden.

What about when you travel? Before I leave home, I research on the Internet to find organic markets and restaurants in the cities Don and I will visit. We will drive many miles to buy fresh, organic food. We have even driven two hours out of our way to have organic, vegetarian meals instead of fast food on the road.

I have also learned to buy, for the most part, fruits grown in this country and in season. I always look to see where fruit is grown, and while I occasionally eat some tropical fruit, such as bananas, mangoes, or pineapple, I will choose Californian fruit over Mexican or Chilean whenever possible. Among the most pesticide-laden fruits are grapes, oranges, and strawberries, so organic versions of these fruits are well worth the premium they command.

Not only is organic food freer of pesticides, but research shows that it contains far more vitamins and minerals than the devitalized food at our local markets. In studies comparing organic and conventionally grown food, vitamin C is consistently higher in organic food, says Dr. Kate Clancy, Director of the Agriculture Policy Project at the Henry Wallace Institute in Washington, D.C. Organic wheat has been shown to have 430 percent more magnesium and 120 percent more calcium than commercial wheat, while organic potatoes have 110 percent more boron, 220 percent more selenium, and 50 percent more magnesium than commercial potatoes. Since my blood workup showed I was woefully low in magnesium, potassium, and selenium, I am grateful I can obtain these minerals in greater abundance in organic food.

Organic food is not only better for our health, but it tastes better too. If you don't believe me, do the taste test. Purchase green beans (or any green vegetable, for that matter) at your local market, and then buy the organic version of the same vegetable. Steam both and taste the difference. That difference is the vitamins and minerals your body desperately needs.

CONSUME NATURE'S SUPERSTARS

As you begin to concentrate on a plant-based diet, you should maximize your intake of the produce "superstars" among our fruits and veggies.

Tomatoes

According to Donna Weihofen, senior nutritionist at the University of Wisconsin Comprehensive Cancer Center, research shows that regular consumption of tomatoes decreases the risk of prostate cancer. Lycopene, a carotenoid, may also decrease prostate tumor size and make prostate cancer less aggressive. Lycopene is so good at mopping up free radicals (those unstable molecules that damage cells, cell membranes, and DNA) that it outperforms beta carotene. Not only does it help ward off prostate cancer, but it is good for breast cancer and cancers of the digestive tract as well. But with tomatoes, cooked is better than fresh because cooking concentrates the amount of available lycopene. Whereas a fresh tomato has four milligrams of lycopene per serving, tomato sauce has twenty-three milligrams, and tomato juice has eighteen milligrams.[10] Since the research suggests that ten servings of cooked tomatoes weekly help prevent prostate cancer, think about a nightly serving of low sodium, organic tomato juice, and the rest is easy.

Dr. Block agrees. However, he points out that "a small amount of fat—preferably good fat from fish, flax, walnuts, or olive oil (omega-9 fatty acids)—is needed to take advantage of lycopene in tomatoes." Recently he is finding clinical benefits from his research on increased lycopene intake that can help reverse prostate cancer. He says, "Even a few weeks of supplementing with tomato extract is enough to shrink prostate tumors, while reducing PSA levels (a marker associated with prostate cancer progression)."[11] You can purchase concentrated tomato extract at your health-food store. Suggested dosage? Thirty milligrams a day divided into two doses.

Cruciferous Vegetables

Among the cruciferous vegetables, broccoli is queen. I don't particularly like broccoli, and the same may be true for you. But since I am committed to eating the veggie superstars, you will always find broccoli and its cruciferous relatives (cabbage, Brussels sprouts, cauliflower, Chinese cabbage, collards, kale, kohlrabi, radishes, turnips, watercress) in my refrigerator. In fact, if you were to open my refrigerator, practically all you would see would be veggies!

Broccoli is loaded with antioxidants (quercetin, glutathione, beta carotene, indoles, vitamin C, lutein, glucarate, sulforaphane). It is especially helpful for those with lung, colon, and breast cancer. In fact, it helps remove estrogen from the body speedily, and its indol-3-carbinol may turn harmful estrogen into a more benign form. Unfortunately, overcooking destroys its cancer-fighting potential, so eat this superstar raw in salads or lightly steamed.[12] My broccoli-hating family loves raw broccoli when combined with sunflower seeds, raisins, and onions in a light soy mayonnaise dressing. Try sautéing broccoli and chopped garlic in a small amount of olive oil for another dish.

Since cabbage also has been found to block colon, breast, and stomach cancer, I try to include raw cabbage in my daily diet. I add it to either salads or juice.

Berries

Blueberries are a wonderful part of any anticancer diet, containing more antioxidants than any other fruit or vegetable. They are rich in phytochemicals called anthocyanins, which combat free-radical damage in the body and protect against heart disease and cancer.[13] You can also enjoy delicious raspberries and strawberries—just skip the ice cream and eat them straight. Raspberries are antiviral and anticancer and, as one oncologist said, promote apoptosis, or cancer-cell death. Strawberries also have both antiviral and anticancer capacity but are, unfortunately, one of the most heavily contaminated fruits in your local market. That's why I will eat only organic strawberries in season. Grow your own, or find someone who will sell you strawberries. I have a friend who has a wonderful organic farm with a raspberry patch and five hundred blueberry plants, so many summer days find me picking berries at the farm and sampling the wares as I go.

Garlic and Onions

In *Food—Your Miracle Medicine*, science writer Jean Carper says that garlic is "an all around wonder drug" that lowers blood pressure; combats bacteria, intestinal parasites, and viruses; lowers cholesterol; and contains multiple cancer-fighting compounds and antioxidants. It is the enemy of stomach cancer, in particular.[14] So how do you eat this smelly rose? To combat cancer, it is best to eat raw, aged, or pickled garlic. Also, chop the garlic, and allow it to sit for about fifteen minutes to release important enzymes before you eat it. Even though it stinks, I wouldn't go through a day without one or two cloves chopped up in my salad. Only once has anyone complained, and that was at a wedding reception. My friend said I smelled like a Yugoslavian train—not nice! I got back at her by telling the whole table what she had said. Boy, was she embarrassed! I now make a special point of brushing my teeth vigorously when going out into polite society after a garlic-heavy meal.

Onions also have anticancer power and are particularly good at combating stomach cancer. They are the richest source of a potent antioxidant, quercetin. Onions thin blood, lower cholesterol, fight asthma and chronic bronchitis, and have antiviral, antibiotic, anti-inflammatory capacity.[15] You can eat your daily half of an onion raw (the preferred way) or put the whole, unpeeled onion in the oven and bake it. Once you peel it, you'll discover it's sweetly delicious.

Whole Grains

If you're a fan of instant cereals or white bread, give up the habit. Begin to reduce your intake of refined carbs and replace them with whole grains: quinoa, wheat berries, spelt, whole wheat, buckwheat, couscous, steel cut oats, brown rice, amaranth, millet, barley, and tabbouleh. Whole grains haven't had all nutrients processed out of them. Granted, you will need to cook these longer than more processed foods, but the nutritional reward is worth it. Whole grains are loaded with vitamin E, the B vitamins, minerals, protein, fiber, and important phytonutrients. Your daily dose of whole grains (with insoluble fiber) and your consumption of fruit (soluble fiber) will promote regularity.

Wheat bran is particularly potent as an anticancer food. According to Jean Carper, wheat bran can suppress polyps in the colon and reduce the amount of estrogen floating around in a woman's body, especially important for postmenopausal women. On the negative side, wheat is associated with allergies.[16] If you think you may be allergic to wheat, try spelt bread or waffles.

For breakfast I usually have cooked or raw oatmeal. I actually prefer it raw and keep a mixture of one cup oats, one cup barley flakes, and a half-cup rye flakes in the refrigerator. I take about a cup of this mixture, add two to three tablespoons of freshly ground flaxseed, a few almonds if I'm not having fruit for lunch, and a few raisins, and pour rice milk or almond milk on it. A bowl of that mix will keep me full until one in the afternoon.

Legumes

Several years ago I heard Dr. John McDougall speak at a conference for vegetarians, and he said the best diet in the world is the Daniel diet, referring to the diet the Old Testament describes Daniel and his Hebrew companions as eating, which made them healthier and ruddier than all the other young men who ate at the king's table—after a mere ten days. The Daniel diet consists of water and vegetables, including pulse or beans, peas, and lentils. Beans are a wonderful addition to your anticancer diet. Lima beans, black beans, lentils, navy beans, kidney beans, white beans, aduki, chickpeas, and pinto beans all contain isoflavones and protease inhibitors.[17]*

At a medical conference I heard master herbalist Dr. James Duke say that beans contain genestein and diadzein, naturally occurring phytoestrogens that may block the action of estrogen, slowing the growth of hormonally dependent tumors. He added that our genes have known beans far longer than the twenty-seven-year-old drug tamoxifen, a drug used to inhibit breast-cancer recurrence. He also prefers black beans to soy because they are less fatty and have not been as heavily processed.[18]

Though I admit I have eaten lots of canned organic beans, it's better to eat unprocessed beans whenever possible. I actually have a wonderful black bean recipe, which I've included in the book, and when I make a pot of these sumptuous black beans, my husband and I have a wonderful addition to salads or one of the basic ingredients of wraps. If you have difficulty digesting beans at first, add them gradually or try the digestive enzyme Beano.

Beans are the perfect high-fiber, low-fat, high-protein food. Since I consume about a 90 percent vegetarian diet, I rely on beans, along with plant protein, for my daily protein. When combined with rice, they provide a complete protein.

---

* All references attributed in the endnotes to this source are from *Herbal Medicine, Healing and Cancer: A Comprehensive Program for Prevention and Treatment* by D. Yance and A. Valentine, © 1999 Keats Publishing, reprinted by permission of The McGraw-Hill Companies.

Soy

While soy is one of the most heavily touted foods in America, particularly since the advent of Dr. Bob Arnot's *The Breast Cancer Prevention Diet,* soy consumption does have its detractors. Dr. Max Gerson did not advocate the consumption of any soy products, including tofu, tempeh, miso, soy protein, or soy milk, when fighting cancer. He stated that soy is high in fat, protein, and sodium and that it inhibits the absorption of certain nutrients.[19] Soy is not only a heavily processed food, but it is also a weak estrogen, and because of this, I have heard some physicians suggest it is not ideal for women who have had breast cancer, particularly the consumption of concentrated soy protein powders.

When I asked Dr. Block about soy, he told me, "The earlier concerns about soy promoting breast cancer have yet to be substantiated. In fact, the opposite seems to be the case. While there may be a small subpopulation of breast-cancer patients who may not benefit from soy consumption, the growing evidence and consensus supports higher soy intake for prostate and breast cancer patients." If you choose to eat soy products, and I do occasionally, fermented soy products like tempeh and tofu are better digested.

Green Superfoods

Early in my dietary changes, I added green superfoods to my daily regimen. Green superfoods—and you'll find a variety of them at your health-food store—are a nutritious source of vitamins and minerals. Some products include Kyo Greens, Green Magma, spirulina, wheat grass, Beyond Greens, and Barley Essence. Barley is an ancient grain that is mentioned in the Bible thirty-seven times.[20] In my research, I learned about a Japanese physician and pharmacologist who had mercury poisoning at age thirty-eight. Attempting to find a cure for his illness, he first tried drugs and megadoses of vitamins, with no success. Then he tried herbal remedies and cleansing fasts, which didn't work either. Finally he regained his health by consuming natural enzymes, raw chlorophyll, natural vitamins and minerals, and amino acids—all contained in a powder of green barley leaves.[21]

I take several tablespoons of powdered green barley leaves daily, and the product I use is Kyo Greens, which also contains wheatgrass (a known tumor inhibitor), kelp, and brown rice. My husband, a healthy sixty-nine-year-old who is never ill, says that this green drink alone has increased his energy level by 30 percent. Dr.

Block told me that Don is not the only one noticing an increase in energy after taking green superfoods. "Similar claims are made by many of my patients," he said. Nearly twenty years ago Block began to experiment with green superfoods using phytochemically rich, organic vegetables juiced in the fields where they were grown. Taking his product, Turbo Greens, is equivalent to consuming one and a half pounds of veggies per day! Block said he found improved vitality and better ability to tolerate chemo and also to detox from toxic metabolites in patients taking green superfoods.

How do you take green superfoods? You buy the powdered green drink in a jar and then mix a tablespoon of it in water. I recommend drinking it when you rise in the morning and then drinking two more glasses thirty minutes before meals, for a total of three green drinks a day. If you don't like the taste when mixed with water, put a tablespoon of the powder in freshly made juice. A plus with the "green drink," as we call it, is that you can take a jar along when you travel and continue getting great nutrition.

THE AMAZING OMEGA-3 OILS

When I was first told by Dr. Shamim to start consuming essential fatty acids because of their cancer-fighting potential, I looked at him blankly. I didn't know what essential fatty acids (EFAs) were. Nor did I know we needed to add them to our diet since our bodies can't produce them. According to Dr. Donald Rudin and Clara Felix in their book *Omega-3 Oils,* our bodies can produce only nonessential fatty acids, yet we require essential fatty acids, found in fish oils and flaxseed, for health. Essential fatty acids are not only important in maintaining the integrity of cell membranes, but they help keep the cell membranes fluid, protecting them from freezing or fracturing. Rudin and Felix state that EFAs help correct prostaglandin imbalances, an important factor in maintaining a strong immune system and fighting cancer.[22]

Omega-6 oils, which are found in corn, safflower, cottonseed, peanut, and sunflower oil, are actual cancer promoters when consumed in excess—increasing tumor formation, size, and number. But those wonderful omega-3 oils, found in cold-water fish, flaxseed, pumpkin seeds, hemp, and walnuts, are beneficial to health. They protect against heart disease as well as cancer. Omega-3 fatty acids also inhibit tumor-cell proliferation and enhance immune function. One study of women with breast cancer found that those whose breast tissue had a high content of alpha linolenic acid (the main omega-3 essential fatty acid) were five times less likely to develop metastases than women whose breast tissue had a low content of essential fatty acids.[23]

Dr. Block told me that an immediate shift to an increased consumption of omega-3 fatty acids is enormously beneficial to anyone struggling with cancer. "The sooner the ratio of good fats to bad fats is reversed, the better chance a cancer patient will have. Think of it this way: Inflammation, platelet stickiness, clotting, resistance to treatment, and cachexia are all associated with cancer progression. Turn around an unhealthy fat ratio to a good one, eating a rich omega-3 diet along with tailored supplementation, and your odds can only improve."

Fish Oil

The two omega-3 superstars are fish oil and flaxseed. Cold-water fish contain two omega-3 fatty acids called DHA and EPA. Since both DHA and EPA are found in our brain cells, synapses, retinas, adrenal and sex glands, cold-water fish rich in omega-3 fatty acids are potentially good for our health and important in cancer prevention.[24]

While some oncologists-nutritionists recommend that cancer patients consume cold-water fish frequently for their omega-3s, my nutritionist suggested that, along with abstaining from all animal products, I wait at least six months before eating cold-water fish. He felt a vegetarian diet gave me the best chance of recovery. I later learned that Dr. Max Gerson suggested his cancer patients postpone eating fish for two years while recovering from their disease, advocating instead the consumption of a vegetarian diet.[25]

If you choose to eat fish, eat fatty fish from clean waters, such as salmon, mackerel, sardines, herring, and blue fish, which are higher in the omega-3s. Do so sparingly and only after you've given your body a chance to heal. And be aware of the potential danger of contamination, even among cold-water fish. The plankton in the oceans has become polluted by industrial and agricultural waste as nickel, mercury, oil, and hydrocyanic acid have been dumped into our coastal waters.[26] These toxins travel up the food chain and become concentrated in the tissues of bigger fish, such as swordfish and tuna. Also, stay away from shellfish. According to Dr. Rex Russell, these garbage collectors of the oceans are loaded with "chemicals, toxins, harmful bacteria, parasites, and viruses."[27] In fact, Dr. Russell told me he'd rather smoke than eat shellfish, which he considers a toxic health hazard.

What about farm-raised fish? A recent article in *USA Today* states that new studies have shown that farm-raised salmon may be more contaminated than wild salmon. A pilot study by Canadian scientist Michael Easton, an expert in ecotoxicology, compared farm-raised and wild salmon and found that while mercury levels were the same, there were ten times more PCBs in farm-raised salmon than in wild salmon. Moreover, pesticide levels were higher in the farm-raised fish.[28]

PCBs and other toxins are concentrated in the pellets that farm-raised salmon eat. Then they are fed antibiotics, treated with pesticide and disinfectants, and given caxthaxanthin to produce their lush pink-tangerine color.[29] Caxthaxanthin is a dye made from petrochemicals, according to the *New York Times,* and without it, farm-raised fish are gray or khaki in color.[30] In addition, farm-raised salmon are packed tightly in tanks or pens, and each pen produces "two metric tons of waste, more waste than a small city produces."[31]

When I asked Dr. Block about the issue of contamination, he said we should be careful how much and which fish we eat due to the presence of pollutants damaging our food supply. However, he did suggest increasing detox foods (garlic, onions, ginger, and the cruciferous veggies) to counter exposure to toxins in the environment.

Whether you eat fish or not, Block suggests you supplement with super high quality nitrogen-packed fish oil capsules that are enterically coated. Take four to six grams a day. Block believes that fish oil capsules "may be among the more important supplements any of us takes." Besides, Block says you would have to eat three ounces of salmon daily just to get enough omega-3s! But he doesn't advise daily fish intake due to contamination concerns. The solution? Add purified fish oil capsules to your diet. "My experience assessing patients' lab data demonstrates there is a need for improved omega-3 levels. Concentrated fish oil is an effective way to favorably change the biochemical environment to achieve a cancer-resistant condition," says Block.

Flaxseed: a Miracle Food

In the past six years I have chosen to rely heavily on flaxseed for my daily EFAs. I tell anyone who will listen that flaxseed is a miracle food. Like the father in *My Big, Fat Greek Wedding* who believes Windex solves all problems, I think flaxseed is a wonder food that most should eat, especially breast-cancer patients. Flaxseed is an excellent source of LNA (alpha linolenic acid); it contains immune-enhancing lignans; and it is a powerful, natural healer that helps to lower cholesterol and, as a physician at NIH told me, is a natural antidepressant. In addition, it promotes tumor regression!

As I researched, I came across references to work being done by Lilian Thompson, Ph.D., at the University of Toronto's Department of Nutritional Medicine. Although she is best known for her animal studies, Dr. Thompson told me she has completed a clinical study on the effects of flaxseed on breast tumors. In her study, the treatment group was given muffins containing two and one-half tablespoons, or twenty-five grams, of ground flaxseed per muffin, while the control group received muffins without flaxseed. After an average of thirty-nine days between diagnosis and surgery, Dr. Thompson found the rate of tumor growth decreased in the treatment group. Apoptosis, or cancer-cell death, occurred as well. When I asked Dr. Thompson what she thought was causing this, she replied, "The lignans in the flaxseed may be binding to the estrogen cell receptor sites in the breast and blocking the estrogen." She added that while this may be one "mechanism" producing the tumor regression and cancer-cell death, "it could also be due to the antioxidants in the flaxseed, the way the lignans influence the enzymes involving estrogen synthesis or the omega-3 fatty acids in flaxseeds."

Dr. Thompson was quick to say that the women in her breast-cancer study were not taking drugs. Concerned about the possibility of flax and drug interaction, Dr. Thompson said that if a woman is taking tamoxifen, she should consult her physician before adding flaxseed to her anticancer protocol. She added, "There's no published data showing adverse health effects if one takes flaxseed with tamoxifen, but one should take both with caution."[32]

This is exciting research. While flaxseed is certainly no substitute for tamoxifen, it shares this one mechanism: Soy, tamoxifen, and flaxseed compete with estrogen at cell receptor sites. And being food, flaxseed has no side effects while doing other positive things for the body.

For the heroes in the crowd, flaxseed oil can be consumed straight. You will need to take one tablespoon of oil for each one hundred pounds of body weight. The oil has to be refrigerated, and when it begins to have a strong taste, toss it and purchase a replacement. But the best way to add flax to your diet is to grind the seeds daily in a coffee grinder and sprinkle them over your whole-grain cereal, use them on salads or a baked potato, or add them to a smoothie. If you prefer to grind the seeds, you will need to consume three to four tablespoons daily (about one-fourth cup). Grind only what you need, and eat it within fifteen minutes because of oxidation. Flax, once ground or turned into an oil, is highly perishable. Because of possible rancidity and loss of potency, don't buy the bags of ground flaxseed at the grocer that have sat on the shelf for days or weeks, and don't try to store your own.

If you are concerned about getting your EFAs and want to find a rich source that, if organically grown, is exempt from contamination, then flaxseed is for you. Johanna Budwig, the German scientist who did early research on EFAs in the fifties, believed that cancer patients suffered from a severe deficiency of EFAs in their blood. She worked with cancer patients, using flaxseed oil as a therapeutic agent, and had astounding results.[33] Aware of her research, Dr. Max Gerson started using flax oil with his cancer patients—the only oil he advocated for his sick patients—and found it improved the results of his cancer therapy. The oil, he believed, "helped carry vitamin A (beta carotene) through the bloodstream to enhance the patient's immune response."[34]

I should add that Dr. Block does not believe flaxseed alone will provide sufficient omega-3 fatty acids for most patients due to differences in enzymatic activity among people. He recommends taking fish oil capsules plus two or more tablespoons of ground flaxseed daily. He prefers ground seeds to oil because the seeds contain lignans.

In a lighter vein, daily consumption of flaxseed has positive cosmetic benefits. Lots of my healthy friends take flaxseed every day for its cosmetic value alone. They don't care about EFAs or flaxseed's cancer-fighting potential (although they should), but they do care about the way they look. They tell me that after several weeks on daily flaxseed, their skin feels softer and more supple, and their hair grows faster and has more body. I can personally testify to the same results.

Although research on flaxseed in humans is in the early stages, researchers in

North America have already discovered the value of flax oil in treating tumors, metastases, inflammatory conditions, diabetes, high triglycerides, and other degenerative diseases. I believe the future will prove that flaxseed is a miracle food for those who are healthy as well as for those who seek to reclaim their health.

Nuts

Although nuts are loaded with fat, the type of fats found in nuts—monounsaturated and polyunsaturated—is considered good fat. Nuts lower blood levels of triglycerides and LDL (the bad cholesterol) while raising HDL (the good cholesterol). Pecans and walnuts contain a phytochemical called ellagic acid, which triggers apoptosis, or cancer-cell death. Nuts also contain lots of vitamin E, an antioxidant.[35] Since it is important to lower fat consumption, particularly in fighting an active cancer, you will want to eat nuts sparingly at first. In recent years Dr. Shamim has advised me to eat ten to fifteen almonds several times a week for their cancer-fighting potential. So while nuts are good for cancer prevention, early on they should be consumed judiciously. Later they can become a regular part of your diet.

If you are a healthy person and are seeking to prevent cancer, then you can consume nuts four to five times a week. Eat only a small handful, and concentrate on almonds and walnuts for their omega-3 capacity. Stay away from peanuts, because they may contain a fungus, aflatoxin, known to be carcinogenic. Say good-bye to peanut butter but hello to an even tastier competitor, almond butter, which provides excellent nutrition. Almond butter is stocked in the same section as peanut and cashew butter in health-food stores. Once you try it, you'll quickly become hooked on its delicate, rich taste.

Forget the roasted, heavily salted varieties of nuts. Instead, always eat nuts raw and unsalted, and keep them in the refrigerator to preserve their freshness.

WATER: THAT LIFE-GIVING FORCE

We have all heard ad nauseam that we should drink eight to ten glasses of water daily. But why is water so important to the body, especially the body that's fighting cancer cells? To begin with, our bodies are 75 percent water and our brains, 85 percent water. In fact, water is needed to regulate all our bodily functions, including the ability of the kidneys to expel toxins from the body.

Yet, ironically, according to an intriguing book titled *Your Body's Many Cries for Water* by F. Batmanghelidj, M.D., most Americans live in a perpetual state of dehydration with bodies constantly in drought management. A lot of pain that we medicate—such as ulcers, heartburn, and headaches—are indications that our bodies are crying out for water. In fact, in a 1987 address given to international cancer researchers, Dr. Batmanghelidj suggested that "chronic dehydration in the human body is a primary causative factor in tumor production."[36]

How can you tell if you're getting enough water? Just do a urine check. Dr. Batmanghelidj suggests that ideally urine should be colorless or pale yellow. If your urine is orange or dark yellow, you're becoming dehydrated. "It means the kidneys are working hard to get rid of toxins in the body in very concentrated urine."[37] And if your urine is dark, then you're really dehydrated.

But what if you seldom get thirsty? Apparently, thirst is not a good indicator of our need for water because the sensation of thirst diminishes as we age. In fact, if we wait until we feel thirsty to drink water, then we are truly dehydrated. Also, many of us think that because we consume other liquids (tea, coffee, juice), we have less need for water. However, coffee, tea, and soft drinks are actually diuretics that cause our bodies to excrete water. Thus, the heavy coffee drinker will actually need to drink more water than average.

So, we must drink water. Lots of it. Not tap water loaded with chlorine and fluoride, pesticides, or microbes, but pure water that comes from a reputable spring or has been distilled. And we need to drink the requisite amount, eight to ten glasses per day. I find it helpful to measure eight glasses of water into a container in the morning so I can keep track visually of how much I still need to drink.

When is the best time to drink water? We should not drink water with meals since this dilutes digestive juices in the intestines. A good rule of thumb is to drink between meals, a half-hour before eating and an hour after eating.

One caution. If you are dehydrated and have been so for years, then rehydrate slowly. "The cells of the body are like sponges; it takes some time before they become better hydrated."[38] And if you have kidney damage, consult your physician before consuming lots more water.

DR. DEAN ORNISH HAS DONE IT AGAIN

At this point, we turn to some exciting research on the power of food in reversing prostate cancer. Dr. Dean Ornish, founder, president, and director of the nonprofit Preventive Medicine Institute in Sausalito, California, and Clinical Professor of Medicine at the University of California in San Francisco, is a revolutionary. In 1990—when other doctors said it couldn't be done—he provided clinical evidence that heart disease could be reversed with lifestyle changes alone. No drugs. No surgery. Now he has completed a study of men with prostate cancer that shows, once again, that diet and lifestyle changes may have the power to affect the progression of disease.

Here's how it happened. Five years ago Dr. Ornish and his colleagues began a study to see how dietary and lifestyle changes could affect the progression of prostate cancer. The rationale for such a study? According to Ornish, "Conventional medical treatment for prostate cancer usually leaves men impotent or incontinent, and little evidence exists to show that such treatment will prolong life." He continued, "Besides, among the cancers, breast, prostate, and colon are the most responsive to diet."

In Dr. Ornish's study, the experimental group of forty-one patients was asked to make both dietary and lifestyle changes, while the control group was free to make changes if they wished. After twelve months Dr. Ornish found that PSA levels dropped 4 percent in the experimental group, while they went up 6 percent in the control group. These differences were statistically significant. He presented these findings in April 2003 at the annual scientific meeting of the American Urological Association in Chicago.

"The diet reduces your intake of disease-promoting substances such as cholesterol, saturated fat, and oxidants and also provides at least a thousand other substances that are protective against disease," said Dr. Ornish. What dietary changes did the participants in the experimental group make? The men ate a vegan diet consisting of fruits, vegetables, beans, grains, and soy. Whereas Dr. Ornish's heart patients were allowed to eat low-fat cheese, the prostate cancer group was asked to avoid dairy altogether. "A Harvard study found that the consumption of dairy may increase the incidence of prostate cancer," Dr. Ornish told me.

In addition, the prostate cancer patients avoided simple carbohydrates (such as sugar, honey, white flour, white rice), which are low in fiber and cause blood sugar to increase rapidly, stimulating the body to produce excessive amounts of insulin. Instead, they ate whole foods or complex carbohydrates (like beans, grains, vegetables, and fruits), which are rich in fiber and are absorbed slowly, helping to keep blood sugar constant.

Dr. Ornish believes that soy may help prevent prostate cancer because its weak phytoestrogens bind to cell receptor sites, helping to keep the bad estrogen out. He did state, however, that soy might not be a good idea for women who are estrogen receptor-positive or who are taking tamoxifen.

In addition to a vegan diet, the experimental group consumed three grams of fish oil daily (from a refrigerated, lightproof bottle) for their essential fatty acids. According to Ornish, "Three grams per day of fish oil provide the essential fatty acids without the excessive fat and mercury that are often present in fish." When I asked about flaxseed, Dr. Ornish said that while flaxseed oil or ground seeds may be a good idea for women with breast cancer, some research has shown that it may worsen prostate cancer.

In addition to dietary changes, the participants in the experimental group were asked to make other significant lifestyle changes. They participated in weekly support groups. "While support groups may or may not prolong life, they do help participants stay on the program and reframe their illness in a more helpful way," he said. In addition, members of the experimental group walked for a half-hour each day and spent an hour doing yoga, meditation, stretching exercises, and deep breathing. "These practices are compatible with whatever religious tradition a patient has," commented Ornish. "We know that chronic stress suppresses the immune function, so this time of relaxation helps quiet the mind and body. Also, these techniques can be profoundly transformative. They help people to quiet down their mind and body in order to experience more of an inner sense of peace and well-being, more in touch with the source of life. They often become less fearful of death."

At the end of our conversation, Dr. Ornish turned reflective. "While no one wants to be diagnosed with prostate cancer or heart disease, suffering can be a powerful catalyst for change. We help people to find ways of living that are life-enhancing rather than self-destructive."[39]

So What's the Bottom Line?

At this point you may be overwhelmed, thinking, *How can I possibly keep track of the juicing, green drinks, and fruits and veggies I need to consume daily?* I felt the same way when I began to transform my diet. Now my routine is easy and simple. To get you started, I've included a "Day in the Life of a Food Hero" to show you how to sequence and simplify your daily regime. Yes, it takes thought and time. But, as Dr. Nicholas Gonzalez, a prominent physician who works with cancer patients, told me, "Nutrition is foundational in any cancer recovery. Only as patients feel better can they work on those other areas of their lives: the psychological and the spiritual."[40] Indeed.

❖ A Day in the Life ❖

To help get you started with a diet- and supplement-based approach to cancer, I've included a daily regimen. While preparing such a large number of fresh juices, salads, and organic meals may seem overwhelming at first, you will quickly get the hang of sequencing food combinations and ensuring that you eat and drink enough fruits and vegetables daily.

Upon Arising

Green drink: one tablespoon of a green drink, such as Kyo Greens or Turbo Greens, dissolved in eight ounces of water

Green tea: a cup of decaf green tea during your time of journal writing, reflection, Bible reading, or prayer

Breakfast (45 minutes later)

Cooked oatmeal or raw muesli (oats, barley, rye flakes, almonds, ground flax) with Rice Dream and spelt toast or whole wheat toast

or

Sliced fresh fruit (such as bananas, grapefruit, apples, oranges, kiwi) and a small handful of almonds or walnuts

or

Cooked millet, Rice Dream, and spelt or whole wheat toast

Midmorning

Eight ounces of fresh vegetable juice (six to eight carrots, a handful of parsley, one or two stalks of celery)

Thirty Minutes Before Lunch

A green drink or another eight-ounce glass of fresh vegetable juice

Lunch

Green salad with seven or more chopped vegetables, organic black beans, and salsa

or

Vegetarian sandwich (hummus, onions, avocado, tomato, sprouts)
on whole-grain bread and salad
or
Fruit lunch with almonds
or
Homemade veggie or lentil soup, salad, and whole-grain bread

Midafternoon
Eight ounces of vegetable juice

Half-Hour Before Dinner
Eight ounces of vegetable juice or green drink or tomato juice

Dinner
Sweet potato, steamed veggies, veggie burger, and salad
or
Wraps (tortillas, hummus, beans, sweet potatoes, sprouts, brown rice,
salsa) and salad
or
Whole-grain pasta, steamed veggies, piece of whole-grain bread,
salad
or
Veggie stir-fry with seitan (a wheat flour product), brown rice,
salad

Between Meals
Everyone should drink at least six to eight glasses of water a day between meals. Don't drink anything with your meal, to ensure proper digestion of your food. And if you have an active cancer, you'll want to drink six to eight glasses of vegetable juice, sequencing them every hour or so. (As you increase your juices, you'll obviously need to reduce water intake or you'll float away!) Remember: Since fruit should be consumed alone, don't mix fruit and veggies when you juice. The only exception is an apple. You may use apples with carrot juice or the juice of fresh greens.

❖   How to Eat Out Without Losing Your Mind   ❖

Don and I have always enjoyed eating out, and we still do. But since I've had cancer, I've learned that in most restaurants it's hard to find anything with nutritional value that hasn't been overcooked, heavily salted, or soaked in oil or butter. These are tips I've learned to protect my health without giving up my social life:

- If I can choose the restaurant, I look for a vegetarian or ethnic one. Japanese, Thai, or Mediterranean (such as Lebanese or Greek) restaurants usually have healthy, vegetarian entrées and may also serve brown rice.

- If I'm meeting a friend at an American restaurant with a decent salad bar, I load up on fresh veggies (no fruit, as the two shouldn't be combined) and beans.

- If there's no salad bar, I'll order a fresh fruit plate or a vegetarian sandwich with the best salad they serve. I get my nonfat dressing on the side and dip my fork in it to reduce my fat intake. Most often, I'll squeeze lemon juice onto my salad and use that as my dressing. Another option is to ask for steamed veggies with no oil or butter. Or I'll scan the menu for anything raw and order that. I avoid restaurant soups, as they typically are made with butter and heavy cream and loaded with salt. Ditto for pasta, which is usually made from white flour.

- If the restaurant has nothing I can eat, and I know it, I'll eat ahead of time. No matter how tasty the food, I simply can't afford to eat high-fat, low-food-value entrées. So I'll prepare my own meal at home and order herbal tea or sparkling water to drink while my friends chow down. I also eat at home before receptions or parties when I know there will be an abundance of high-fat appetizers or sweets and little else.

The good news? Most restaurants now serve at least one vegetarian entrée for the growing number of customers who are seeking to control their diets for health or personal reasons. If you look at a menu and can't find anything to eat, don't be afraid to ask the waiter if the chef will prepare a special meal. Most restaurants will try to accommodate patrons by reducing oils and fats, serving dressings on the side, or modifying entrées.

My favorite restaurants by far are the funky vegetarian establishments we have discovered in our travels. Don and I will often drive an hour or so out of our way to have a delicious meal at one of our favorite vegetarian hot spots. Among our favorites: The Manatee Café, south of Jacksonville, Florida, which has great burritos, salads, and tofu pumpkin pie, and Blind Faith in Evanston, Illinois, which has delicious entrées. Here are some tips for finding new haunts:

- Don't be put off by the restaurant's exterior. Many organic vegetarian restaurants have a minimalist style or are painted funky colors, but inside a dedicated culinary artist is working hard in the kitchen.

- Always carry food in a cooler when you travel. That way you don't have to succumb to fast food when you're starving. A recent article in the *USA Today* travel section titled "Cheap but Chic" said that so many Americans now travel with coolers that it's become hip. Don and I usually pack ours with almond butter, spelt bread, fruit, carrots, celery, and hummus veggie sandwiches.

- Learn to eat at health-food stores. Most have tasty entrées, good vegan soups, delicious whole-grain bread, and excellent organic salad bars. Eating at a grocery store is neither exciting nor romantic, but the food is generally nutritious. Whole Foods, Wild Oats, and Earth Fare are several of the national and regional chains where you can buy inexpensive, delicious food. Just remember that organic prepared food can be high-fat, too: Just because it's freshly made, doesn't mean it isn't packed with unnecessary calories and cream, butter, and oil. So choose wisely, read labels, and ask the staff about deli and prepared foods to ensure that you're eating healthfully.

"Seafood" Salad
from Hippocrates' Executive Chef Kelly Serbonich[41]

2 cups sea vegetables
   of your choice*

1 cup celery, thinly sliced

1 cup carrots, shredded

¼ cup onion, diced

1 cup fresh parsley, chopped

½ cup pine nuts, soaked in water

1 tablespoon fresh lemon juice

1 clove garlic

4 drops liquid stevia extract

¼ teaspoon ground turmeric

1 teaspoon ground mustard seed

cayenne to taste

water as needed to blend

Braggs aminos, dulse, or kelp
   granules to taste (optional)

1. In a mixing bowl, combine the sea vegetables, carrots, celery, onion, and parsley.

2. In a blender, combine the pine nuts, lemon juice, garlic, stevia, turmeric, mustard, cayenne, water, and the flavor enhancer of your choice. Season to taste and adjust the consistency of the dressing using water.

3. Combine the dressing and salad mixture. Let stand at least 30 minutes before serving. Yields 2 servings.

* Sea vegetables are harvested from the ocean and are a rich source of vitamins and minerals.

Avocado Rainbow
from Hippocrates' Executive Chef Kelly Serbonich

1-2 large avocados, diced

1 cup red cabbage, diced

½ cup snow peas

¼ carrot, shredded

½ golden beet, shredded

¼ red onion, diced

¼ red bell pepper, diced

½ bunch fresh basil, chiffonnade

1 clove garlic, pressed

fresh lemon juice to taste

Braggs aminos, dulse, or kelp
   granules to taste (optional)

Mix all ingredients together in a bowl and season to taste. Serve. Yields 2 servings.

Nutty Lentil Salad
from A Banquet of Health by Penny Block[42]

3 cups water

1 cup red lentils, rinsed and drained

1 large yellow onion, minced

1 strip kombu (a sea vegetable)

1 bay leaf

1 clove garlic, minced

¼ teaspoon cumin

6 tablespoons olive oil

3 tablespoons fresh lemon juice

1 teaspoon sea salt

4 green onions, minced

1 stalk celery, chopped

½ cup chopped walnuts (optional)

Bring water to a boil in a large soup pot over high heat. Stir in lentils, yellow onion, kombu, bay leaf, garlic, and cumin; cover and reduce heat to low. Simmer 30 minutes or until lentils are tender. Drain off any excess liquid; remove kombu and bay leaf. Let cool to room temperature; place in large serving bowl.

In a small bowl, whisk together olive oil, lemon juice, and salt; pour over lentil mixture. Add green onions and walnuts; toss lightly. Serve warm or chilled.

Variation: **Cilantro-Lentil Salad.** Substitute ¼ cup chopped fresh cilantro for the walnuts.

Pumpkin Seed Hummus
from Hippocrates' Executive Chef Kelly Serbonich

2 ½ cups pumpkin seeds, soaked in water

1 clove garlic

1 tablespoon fresh lemon juice

1 tablespoon ground cumin

2 teaspoons ground coriander

¼ cup extra virgin olive oil

2-3 drops liquid stevia extract

Braggs aminos, dulse, or kelp granules to taste (optional)

In a food processor, combine all ingredients. Process until smooth. Add liquid if necessary to process. Season to taste. Serve with vegetable sticks or chips. Yields 3 cups.

Seitan Stroganoff
from A Banquet of Health by Penny Block

1 large onion, chopped

canola or olive oil

2 cloves garlic, crushed

1 teaspoon sea salt

6 ounces silken tofu, puréed

3-4 tablespoons sake (optional)

2 tablespoons shoyu

10-12 mushrooms, sliced

2-3 cups seitan, cut into ¼-inch strips

¼ teaspoon dried basil

2 tablespoons chopped fresh parsley

Lightly coat the bottom of a large skillet with oil; place over high heat. Sauté onion 3 to 4 minutes or until translucent. Stir in garlic; sprinkle with salt. Stir in tofu; cook 2 to 3 minutes. Stir in sake and shoyu until well blended. Remove from heat.

Lightly coat the bottom of another large skillet with oil; place over high heat. Sauté mushrooms 3 to 4 minutes until they just begin to brown. Stir in seitan. Cook, covered, over low heat until mushrooms are tender. Stir in basil. Pour tofu mixture over seitan-mushroom mixture; simmer 3 to 4 minutes. Serve hot over cooked soba or rice; garnish with parsley.

Black Bean Soup
from my friend Jane Graham

1 pound black beans

1 large onion, chopped

6 cloves garlic, chopped

½ red bell pepper

½ yellow bell pepper

  (or 1 whole green pepper)

2 tablespoons vinegar

2 bay leaves

1 tablespoon cumin

2 teaspoons oregano

At the last add salt and pepper.

Cover beans with water and bring to a boil. Turn off the heat, cover, and let the beans sit for 1 hour. Drain, rinse, and cover with water. Sauté the onion, garlic, and peppers, and add to the beans, along with the seasonings and vinegar. Cook until the beans are tender. Then serve over rice. They are especially good on brown rice.

Italian Quinoa Salad
from A Banquet of Health by Penny Block

3 cups cooked quinoa,*
  at room temperature

4 green onions, chopped

½ cup chopped fresh fennel
  (bulbs and fronds)

½ red bell pepper, cored, seeded,
  and chopped

⅓ cup sliced black olives (optional)

3 tablespoons minced fresh parsley

2-3 tablespoons olive oil

1½ tablespoons balsamic vinegar

1 pinch sea salt, or to taste

1 pinch black pepper, or to taste
kale leaves (optional)

Combine quinoa, green onions, fennel, bell pepper, olives (if desired), and parsley in large serving bowl; toss lightly.

Whisk together oil, vinegar, salt, and black pepper; pour over quinoa-vegetable mixture. Toss lightly; refrigerate. Serve chilled, mounded on steamed kale leaves, if desired.

* Quinoa (KEEN wa) is an ancient grain, richer in protein than other grains. It also contains the amino acid lysine, calcium, vitamin E, and B complex.

Shredded Brussels Sprouts
from A Banquet of Health by Penny Block

½ pound Brussels sprouts, rinsed and trimmed

olive oil

¼ teaspoon sea salt

1 tablespoon fresh lime juice or balsamic vinegar

¼ teaspoon garlic powder

1 pinch black pepper

1 teaspoon water

Shred Brussels sprouts by thinly slicing lengthwise into small pieces. Lightly coat the bottom of the skillet with oil; place over medium heat. Sauté Brussels sprouts 3 minutes; sprinkle with salt. Stir in lime juice, garlic powder, and pepper; sauté 2 minutes. Sprinkle with water; cover and steam 2 minutes. Serve hot.

Imperial Tofu Salad
from The Laughing Seed Café[43]

As most people who eat tofu have discovered, there are secrets to making it taste really good. The executive chef at The Laughing Seed Café knows most of those secrets, as this recipe demonstrates. Try it in a sandwich or as a replacement for chicken salad. It's also great with chips or pita, mounded on a salad, or even on toast with a slather of white miso or avocado.

Here's the secret for the tofu:

Dice 1 pound of tofu in half-inch cubes. Toss gently with enough olive oil to lightly coat the cubes. Add salt and pepper to taste and enough curry powder to turn the tofu a light yellow. Bake on a cookie sheet 30-40 minutes at 350 degrees, depending on the size of your cubes. This will give the tofu a chewy, meaty quality. Remove from oven before tofu begins to harden. This method of cooking tofu can be used in many recipes. Larger cubes are great for kabobs, stir-fries, or in Indian dishes to replace paneer.

Cool tofu before adding:

1 stalk celery, finely diced

3 scallions, chopped

½ red bell pepper, finely diced

In a blender or a food processor:

¾ cup soy mayonnaise

1 teaspoon rice vinegar

1 teaspoon Dijon mustard

1 teaspoon tamari

1 tablespoon tahini

In a food processor grind:

¼ cup sunflower seeds

⅛ cup pumpkin seeds

⅛ cup sesame seeds

½ teaspoon lemon juice

1 clove garlic, chopped

Add Modern Food Products "Spike" to taste.

Mix all ingredients and chill before serving.

Veggie Pita
from The Manatee Café[44]

Take ½ pita. Add sliced tomato, sliced onions, raw shredded cabbage, sliced mushrooms, shredded carrots, cooked sweet potato, chopped broccoli, avocado, cooked cabbage, salsa, soy cheese (optional), and a low-fat, low-sodium dressing. Put in the oven for 3-5 minutes. Then add sprouts.

Banana Cream Pie
from Hippocrates' Executive Chef Kelly Serbonich

3 cups walnuts, soaked and dehydrated

½ teaspoon Braggs liquid aminos

¼ cup dates, pitted and soaked

2 cups young coconut meat

3 medium-ripe bananas, broken into pieces

2 tablespoons alcohol-free vanilla extract

⅔ cup macadamia nuts, soaked in water

10 dates, pitted and soaked

½ cup young coconut water

1 teaspoon psyllium husks powder

4 ripe bananas, sliced

For the crust: Using a food processor, finely grind the walnuts to a crumble. Add the 4-5 dates and Braggs aminos and process until combined. The mixture should be slightly sticky. Press the dough into a pie plate. Dehydrate overnight if a crunchy crust is desired.

For the filling: In a strong blender, combine the coconut meat, 3 bananas, vanilla, macadamia nuts, 10 dates, coconut water, and psyllium powder. Blend until very smooth and creamy. Stir in the sliced ripe bananas and spread evenly over the crust. Chill and serve. Yields 1 pie.

Stir-Fry
from The Manatee Café

A handful of each of the following, chopped:

mushrooms	kale
onions	salsa
broccoli	avocado
carrots	red cabbage
tomatoes	

Sauté all the ingredients together until tender. Add a handful of cooked beans and rice. You may also add tamari or Braggs liquid aminos to taste. Yields 2 cups.

Dragon Plate
from The Laughing Seed Café

This salad features primarily living and enzymatic foods to aid digestion. The Laughing Seed starts with a bed of organic mixed greens and places a scoop of brown rice, soba, or udon noodles in the center of the plate. Ring the rice or pasta with little piles of vegetables, including:

grated carrot

grated red cabbage

diced cucumbers

diced red or yellow tomatoes or cherry tomatoes

diced red and green peppers

clover sprouts

sea vegetable salad

avocado

sauerkraut or pickled daikon

pickled onions

chopped broccoli and cauliflower

top with sunflower and pumpkin seeds

Pickled onions are a delicious accompaniment to rice and vegetable dishes, Indian food, salads, and wraps, and keep in the fridge for days. Our recipe couldn't be easier. Take as many white or yellow onions as you like, slice, then cut slices into halves or quarters. Cover with even amounts of cider vinegar and tamari. Refrigerate for 6 hours before serving.

Veggie Burrito
from The Manatee Café

Take a whole wheat tortilla and add soy cheese, avocado, and salsa. Place on griddle and allow to brown. In a pan add oil and heat until smoking. Add ½ handful of cooked beans and ½ handful of cooked rice with a teaspoon of tamari. Sauté 2 minutes. Put tortilla in oven approximately 1½ minutes. Add beans and rice mix to tortilla. Add sprouts. Fold and cut in half. Serve with blue corn chips and tabbouleh.

Juicing for Life

Juicing is an excellent means of adding fruits and vegetables to your diet. Since juice contains the whole fruit or vegetable—except the fiber—which is the indigestible part of the plant—it contains virtually all of the plant's health-promoting components.

James F. Balch, M.D., and Phyllis A. Balch

Juicing is a wonderful and easy way to absorb a concentrated form of fresh fruits and vegetables. Many cancer clinics around the world use juice therapy as part of their treatment programs.

Donald R. Yance Jr.

Diagnosed with stage 4 breast cancer, Anne Frähm was told by her oncologist that she would be dead within two years. She later learned he was being highly optimistic. Earlier checkups had not caught the cancer before it literally ate a stress fracture into her backbone, causing crippling back pain. After a harrowing protocol—a mastectomy, chemotherapy, hormonal therapy, and a bone marrow transplant—the doctors sent her home to die. Cancer still pervaded her bone marrow, and the doctors were unwilling to enroll her in experimental trials. As Frähm recounted in her book, *Cancer Battle Plan,* she had exhausted all her medical options.

Yet five weeks later, medical tests showed that she had no trace of cancer. According to Frähm, her oncologist was "flabbergasted." "I honestly thought you were doomed," he told her.[1] How was she able to create such a dramatic turnaround? With a strict nutritional regimen that used juicing to detoxify and refortify her body. Frähm embarked on a fourteen-day juice fast to cleanse her body, ingesting vast quantities of carrot juice, apple juice, distilled water, and green drinks, supplemented by megadoses of vitamin C and other supplements. In addition, she detoxified her body with liver cleansing and coffee enemas. Plucky Anne Frähm lived for more than ten years postdiagnosis, and her helpful and optimistic book was the first I read after my own diagnosis.

The success of Frähm's regimen was not accidental; juicing is an integral part of cancer survival for many people, and its importance cannot be overstated. The late Dr. Norman Walker, who lived well past a hundred and created the first, albeit primitive, juicer in America, wrote years ago, "The juices extracted from fresh raw fruits and vegetables form the means of furnishing all the cells in the body with the elements they need, in the manner in which they can be most readily assimilated."[2] Fresh juices are absorbed within ten to fifteen minutes and take minimal effort to digest, allowing our bodies to benefit quickly and easily from this living nutrition. Therefore, juicing allows our bodies to get almost immediate nourishment from living enzymes, which regenerate cells, tissues, glands, and organs in our bodies.

According to Dr. Walker, heating food above 118 degrees destroys vital, life-giving enzymes, while eating only raw foods fails to provide our bodies with adequate nutrition. Not only does it take up to five hours to digest raw food, but much of the raw foods' nourishment is used up during the digestive process, leaving only a "small percentage available for the regeneration of cells and tissues."[3] Juicing is the missing link, giving us the goodness of raw food in its most easily digestible form.

While fruit juices cleanse the body, vegetable juices, according to Dr. Walker, build and regenerate the body. In his book *Fresh Vegetable and Fruit Juices,* originally published in 1936 and reissued every year since, Dr. Walker stated that vegetable juices "contain all the amino acids, minerals, salts, enzymes and vitamins needed by the human body, provided that they are used fresh, raw, and without preservatives, and that they have been properly extracted from the vegetables."[4]

Juicing is a must, not only for those trying to recover from cancer but for those who want to prevent cancer as well. In his book *Dr. Gaynor's Cancer Prevention Program,* Dr. Mitchell Gaynor says that every morning after working out, he goes to a local coffee shop to pick up a glass of juice that has been prepared especially for him. His recipe: two carrots, two stalks of celery, one beet, a bunch of watercress, a third of a cucumber, and half of an apple. He calls this his "phytonutrient power drink."[5] Then it's on to work for this cancer doctor.

Not only does juicing provide our bodies with living enzymes and optimal nutrition, but the juices help flush out the colon to keep us regular. One of my friends who had struggled with constipation for over twenty years told me that drinking a pint of carrot juice daily has changed her life. She no longer has problems with constipation, and because of this, she feels better and more energetic than she has in years.

The Gerson Therapy

So how much fresh juice should you consume daily if you are battling cancer? The late Dr. Max Gerson believed that those who are ill need to consume thirteen eight-ounce glasses of freshly made organic carrot-apple and green veggie juices every day. Charlotte Gerson and Dr. Morton Walker write in *The Gerson Therapy:*

> Along with providing sufficient fluid intake, fresh juices furnish nearly all
> of the nutrients—vitamins, minerals, enzymes, phytochemicals, herbals and
> other food substances, including even proteins—required for your body to
> heal itself. Juice drinking is even more important for healing degenerative
> diseases than eating the same nutrients in whole food.… Juice drinking
> allows for better digestion and greater absorption.[6]

At the Gerson clinic in Tijuana, Mexico, where Charlotte Gerson continues her father's work, patients begin the day with a glass of orange juice, followed by eight glasses of carrot or carrot-apple juice (apples are the only fruit that should be mixed with vegetables), then by four glasses of "green leaf juice." For the "green leaf juice" the clinic suggests mixing such vegetables as romaine or red lettuce, escarole, endive, green pepper, watercress, Swiss chard, beet tops, or red cabbage with a single apple.[7] Each day patients consume thirteen eight-ounce glasses of juice, one hourly, plus three vegetarian meals, which provide the equivalent of seventeen to twenty pounds of life-giving food a day, more than anyone could possibly eat. By drinking all these juices, cancer patients literally flood their bodies with massive amounts of nutrients. This high-quality concentration not only helps the body eliminate toxins, stimulates the metabolism, and increases the availability of oxygen in the blood, but *The Gerson Therapy* suggests that while chemotherapy "boasts an overall remission rate on average of 12 percent," the "Gerson therapy offers total remission success on average for up to 42 percent of its participating largely terminal cancer patients."[8] That's pretty impressive!

YES, YOU CAN!

Drinking thirteen glasses of vegetable juice a day may sound like a daunting assignment, but drinking as much raw vegetable juice as you can is a must if you have an active cancer. In fact, after you eliminate the food villains and begin your vegetarian diet, drinking fresh juice is perhaps the single best thing you can do for your body. Preparing the juice takes only five to ten minutes and is so simple that even my six-year-old grandson can do it! You need to incorporate fresh juice into your everyday life, even if you are ill, pressed for time, or on the road. Here are some strategies for making that happen.

If You Are Ill

Ask family members to take over some—or all—of the juice preparation. A system of daily shifts could split up the responsibility. If you are married, your husband or wife might sign up for before-breakfast duty, while an older child might make the predinnertime juice drink. If this is not an option, consider hiring someone to come every day to make juice for you. Dr. Lorraine Day, who nearly died from recurring breast cancer, said she was so weak when she implemented the Gerson Therapy that she had to hire someone to come to her home every day and make the thirteen glasses of juice for her. Alive and active nine years later, she still consumes eight glasses of vegetable juice daily.

If You Have Limited Time at Home

I suggest the following:
- Drink your fresh juice before breakfast and dinner.
- Find an organic juice bar near work, and go there for lunch, for a quick pit stop during the day, or on the way home.
- Take a thermos of juice to work, and drink from it during the day.

My friend Bob, an eleven-year survivor of bladder cancer, drinks a couple of glasses of fresh juice before he goes to work and then takes the rest of his daily quota in a thermos. Fortunately, Bob's wife is committed to helping him. In fact, Joan cleans and juices twelve or thirteen different vegetables every morning before she heads out to her full-time job. For Bob, all the juicing plus a vegan diet have paid tremendous dividends; he says he feels great and has lots of energy.

If You Are Traveling

Getting fresh juice may be more difficult when you travel, but it is not impossible. I've made it work wherever I've been: cruise ships, trains, motels. You name it, I've juiced there. My motto: *Have juicer, will travel.*

Don and I have carried coolers containing raw veggies into narrow train compartments and watched scenery fly by as we pulverized fat organic carrots, celery, and chard into enzyme-rich juice. (Yes, there was an electrical outlet.) And I may be the only person who has ever juiced raw vegetables on a cruise ship. Several years ago Don and I decided to celebrate our twenty-fourth anniversary by taking our first cruise. While I was excited about seeing the eastern Caribbean, I knew the trip could be lethal to my diet. Since I didn't want to jeopardize my health for this vacation, I packed my Champion juicer and bought twenty pounds of carrots, three bunches of celery, and a bag of apples at the local health-food store in Fort Lauderdale. Don and I then boarded the *Westerdam,* hoisting luggage, bags of raw veggies, a cooler, and juicer, while other passengers casually pulled a single piece of luggage.

Before I travel to a new city, I do my research. I usually locate a health-food store or Whole Foods Market there and, if necessary, will make late-night grocery store runs to stock up on supplies. Through this process, I've become well acquainted with juice bars and vegetarian restaurants up and down the Eastern seaboard. From New York City all the way to Fort Lauderdale, Don and I have mapped out the best places to eat and drink fresh juice. Even now, as I'm dreaming about a trip to Europe, I'm researching which juicer to buy in Germany.

My point? When you make something a high priority, all things are possible. What's most important is to change your mind-set from viewing juicing as optional and a chore to being absolutely critical in your battle against cancer.

WHAT IF YOU HAVE HAD CHEMOTHERAPY?

Chemotherapy patients can benefit from juicing but need to be careful how much they ingest. Charlotte Gerson and Morton Walker suggest that those who have undergone chemotherapy should consume *greatly* reduced amounts of freshly made juice daily. They write: "Pursuing the full, unmodified Gerson protocol for any patient who has undergone chemotherapy, regardless of the time elapsed since the last treatment, can be extremely dangerous."[9] Why is this so? Because the toxic chemicals used for the chemotherapy accumulate in the body. As a consequence, when people begin juicing, healing crises, sometimes severe, can occur. When we begin juicing, our tissues release "accumulated toxins into the bloodstream."[10] While our livers filter out toxins, too much burden on the liver can be dangerous. That's why coffee enemas, which help the liver, are an essential part of the Gerson Therapy.

Gerson and Walker suggest that people who have had chemotherapy start with only two to four ounces of freshly squeezed vegetable or fruit juice at a time and avoid carrot juice. If the juice is well tolerated over a period of days, the cancer patient may slowly increase the juice consumption, adding carrots to the mix after seven to ten days. While Gerson and Walker note that it is possible to rebuild the body after chemotherapy, they have learned from patients who have come to the clinic in Mexico that it is important to proceed slowly with the juicing and other elements of the Gerson Therapy. For more instruction, I recommend you read *The Gerson Therapy.*

The Gersons share the example of a forty-six-year-old woman with metastasized breast cancer, whom they call F. C. With a grim prognosis—cancer had spread to her lungs and infiltrated fourteen of fifteen surgically removed lymph nodes—F. C. embarked on a year-long course of chemotherapy. After nine treatments she was forced to stop. Each treatment had landed her in the hospital with pneumonia or another infection, and her situation was critical. Finally she was sent home with a terminal diagnosis.

With the help of a naturopath, F. C. embarked on the Gerson Therapy but continued to experience nausea and vomiting for several months as she detoxified her body. However, early x-rays encouraged her: Just three weeks into the protocol, the breast and lung cancer growth had stopped, and the tumors were static. Eight months later she finally started to feel better, and at the year mark, she reported, "My skin is glowing, my memory is improved, my hair has grown back thick, and it shows beautiful texture without conditioner."[11] At the time Gerson's book was written, F. C. was twenty-six months into the Gerson Therapy and doing well, even though she continued to have healing crises. The story illustrates the point that while it may take longer to regain one's health after chemo, it is possible to do so.

THE TEN COMMANDMENTS OF JUICING

Here are some tips to help you incorporate juicing into your daily routine:

1. *Buy a good juicer.* I own a sturdy Champion juicer, which typically retails for $200 to $250. This industrial-strength juicer produces nutrient-rich juice, using mastication to pulverize vegetables. Cheaper models fail to extract the fruits and vegetables effectively, leaving most of the nutrients in the pulp. A heavy-duty juicer, the Champion will last for years, given the proper care. Other similar juicers include the Green Power and the Royal, costing $225 to $700.

   Dr. Gerson recommended a more expensive model, the triturator–grinder press combination, as the best. Manufactured by the Norwalk Juicer Sales and Service Company and the K&K Company, this type of juicer extracts maximal enzymes and produces up to a third more juice from the pulp.[12] However, the price tag for this type of juicer—$800 to $2,100—is prohibitive for many families.

   Most people buy a centrifugal juicer, the least expensive of the juicers but also the least effective. Not only does it fail to grind the produce finely enough, but the juice produced by this kind of juicer has fewer healing enzymes, minerals, and phytochemicals than the juice from a masticating juicer and significantly fewer than the juice from the triturator–grinder press combination.

2. *Drink thirteen eight-ounce glasses of juice a day.* If you have cancer, ideally you should juice hourly, drinking thirteen glasses a day—for months. If you can't do that, juice as often as possible, and set a minimum below which you will not go: either a quart or a quart and a half daily, plus green drinks.

3. *Use a variety of fresh, organic vegetables.* With organic produce you eliminate the pesticides and herbicides from your juices. Using carrots as your base, add vegetables like kale, chard, purple cabbage, parsley, cucumbers, beets, and romaine lettuce to the mix. Try different combinations to see which you like best. I've included some recipes at the end of the chapter, but you can also buy juice recipe books.

4. *Drink eight ounces at each juicing.* If the taste is too strong or sweet, dilute the juice by a third with water. Drink the juice slowly; don't gulp it.

5. *Drink the juice immediately after making it* to get the full benefit of all those fabulous living enzymes. Since enzymes die within approximately thirty minutes, it's best if the juice is made fresh before each consumption. But if you can't do this—if you have to take your juice to work in a thermos—you still can get valuable nutrition from juice made hours earlier and refrigerated.

6. *Clean the juicer immediately after using it.* Otherwise the pulp will dry on the attachments and be harder to remove.

7. *Get the family to buy into your new juicing lifestyle.* Explain the importance of juicing, and enlist their practical support. Set up a juicing schedule, and pass the workload around. Encourage your family to drink fresh juice with you; your kids and spouse will probably be more helpful if they also drink the juice.

8. *Take your juicer with you when you travel, and use it.* If you stay with friends or family, explain your situation beforehand and ask to use their kitchen. Explain that you'll clean up each time so that your hosts won't panic when you start spraying vegetables in their kitchen sink. And offer to share your juice. I have friends who line up around my juicer for their freshly made sample, smacking their lips and exclaiming, "This is delicious!"

9. *Do Web or phone research before booking trips to locate the local juice bars.* If possible, start and end each day there. If you have business dinners, make sure you get your fresh juice first.

10. *Use premade and pasteurized juice only as a last resort.* Remember: Pasteurization destroys enzymes. Avoid canned juice since it is enzyme-dead and loaded with sodium and sugar.

READY TO JUICE?

I've included a few recipes to get you started, but your juicer handbook and specialty cookbooks will have other good ideas:

Brenda's Favorites (one pint)
6-8 large carrots
1 small beet
2-3 stalks of celery
small piece of ginger
    or
6-8 large carrots
a handful of parsley
2-3 stalks of celery
    or
6-8 large carrots
a wedge of purple cabbage
2 stalks of Swiss chard

Hippocrates Green Drink (yields 2 cups)
1 ½ cucumbers
4 cups sunflower and buckwheat sprouts
2-3 celery stalks[13]

THE PROOF IS IN THE RESULTS

Juicing will pay great dividends for your investment of time and energy. In the short term, you'll experience increased energy, moister and clearer skin with better texture, freedom from constipation, and a sense of well-being. Longer term, juicing will provide vital nutrients to your body, bolstering your immune system and helping you reclaim your health. As you commit to juicing, you'll be amazed at what this simple but effective protocol will do for your health. Juice on!

Detox Your Way
to Health

*A coffee what? An enema?… How gross! How weird! How sordid! But
on the contrary, how healing and life-saving. And for some it is the difference between life and death.*

SHERRY A. ROGERS, M.D.

T hey'd have to knock me unconscious before I'd give up my coffee enemas,"
said Dr. Nicholas Gonzalez at the end of our interview early one evening.[1]
I thought, *Is this man crazed or what?*

A graduate of Cornell Medical School, Dr. Gonzalez has an office off Park
Avenue in New York City and has worked with over a thousand cancer patients.
The New Yorker calls him "the medical outlaw who is suddenly in demand." Gonzalez's program has received increasing public attention, and the National Insti-
tutes of Health awarded him a $1.4 million grant to conduct a study with
individuals suffering from advanced pancreatic cancer, comparing his enzyme-
nutritional therapy with the best chemotherapy available.[2] His study is "up and
running" and is being carried out by the Columbia College of Physicians and Surgeons, "turning it into the most significant investigation of unconventional cancer
treatment yet sanctioned by the federal government."[3]

While Dr. Gonzalez's program is nutritionally based and requires his patients
to take about 150 pills a day (vitamins, antioxidants, trace minerals, and pancreatic
enzymes), the cornerstone of his program is detoxification. And the primary technique he uses for detoxification is none other than coffee enemas. Why are coffee
enemas essential in detoxing tumor-laden bodies? Gonzalez believes that coffee
enemas not only clean out the lower twelve inches of the colon but also help the

liver function better. Gonzalez told me, "This is critical since the liver is the main detoxification organ in trying to get rid of disease, particularly in 2002 with all the pollution." Gonzalez continued, "When patients start getting better, they're going to dump loads of toxic junk stored in their bodies—heavy metals, pesticides from twenty years ago, food additives. On any good healing program, that stuff is going to start coming out, and patients can get pretty sick unless they take coffee enemas, which really help neutralize, mobilize, and get rid of all that garbage pretty effectively." Because detoxification is so critical, Gonzalez prescribes coffee enemas twice a day for his cancer patients.

But it's not just the sick who benefit from this protocol. Gonzalez takes the "medicine" he prescribes for his patients, taking "almost a hundred pills daily" himself. In addition, he self-administers coffee enemas twice a day. This doctor, whose father died of cancer when Gonzalez was in college, said he adheres to this rigorous regimen not because he has cancer, but because he wants to prevent it.

Michael Specter writes in *The New Yorker* that Gonzalez's use of coffee enemas as a strategic part of detoxification has earned him ridicule from his colleagues. According to Specter, "Gonzalez is fully aware that the enemas are a source of hilarity, disbelief and even outrage."[4] Yet Gonzalez told Specter that not only were coffee enemas possibly used by Florence Nightingale on the battlefields of Crimea, but until the 1970s *The Merck Manual of Diagnosis and Therapy,* a compendium of orthodox therapies and the "medical doctors' therapeutic bible," listed coffee enemas as a legitimate medical treatment. He even tracked down nursing textbooks from the early twentieth century through the 1950s that included coffee enemas as standard therapeutic treatment. Gonzalez said, "No one understood how they worked; they simply made people feel better."

"In my opinion, and I come out of a very orthodox training background, coffee enemas are among the...most important healing remedies on earth," said Gonzalez. "I've been doing them for twenty years, and they have changed my life. I never could drink coffee because it gave me such a terrible feeling, like an anaphylactic reaction. It made me sick. Then I did a coffee enema, and to my astonishment, it made me feel better from day one. Here's where I agree with Gerson, who said about fifty years ago that coffee enemas make the liver work better, and indeed they seem to."

GERSON AND COFFEE ENEMAS

As Gonzalez indicated, one of the most famous physicians to use coffee enemas in treating cancer patients was the late Dr. Max Gerson, who used nutrition to treat Albert Schweitzer's wife, Helene, for tuberculosis, and her recovery was complete. The future healer was born in Wongrowitz, Germany, in 1881, as one of nine children. After his medical training, in 1928 Gerson began treating hopelessly ill cancer patients with a nutritional program he developed to cure his debilitating migraines. His healing diet: fresh fruits and vegetables, mostly raw, and absolutely no salt. Many of his cancer patients who adopted his diet recovered. After immigrating to the United States to escape a Nazi death camp, this Jewish physician opened an office on Park Avenue, where he continued to develop his healing approach to disease, focusing heavily on nutrition and detoxification.[5] Gerson came to believe that coffee enemas are absolutely essential in detoxifying the cancerous body, and at his clinic his patients self-administered coffee enemas as often as every four hours.

In *The Gerson Therapy*, Gerson's daughter, Charlotte Gerson, and Dr. Morton Walker say Dr. Gerson found that cellular systems and body tissues "excreted waste products accumulated over many years from the taking in of poor air, bad water, food additives, viruses, germs, and other toxic items. In order not to overload the liver, which filters these poisons out of the blood, Gerson found a way to open the bile ducts and help the liver to release the body's accumulated poisons by means of his renowned coffee enemas."[6]

Like Gonzalez, Gerson discovered that when patients started to improve, their whole system could be poisoned if they did not have a way to get rid of the "toxic load escaping from all the dysfunctional cells." He found that prescribing coffee enemas every four hours significantly helped his terminally ill cancer patients, who reported additional benefits as well: pain relief, decreased blood pressure, and high fevers that helped destroy tumors. Gerson and Walker write: "The most aggressive kinds of malignancies—melanomas, ovarian cancers, small-cell lung cancers, aggressive lymphomas—retreat the most rapidly. One can almost watch them melt away. Other, less aggressive tumors grow more slowly and retreat less rapidly: the adenocarcinomas (breast cancer, prostate cancer, bone metastases, etc.) disappear slowly but steadily. At the same time, the fat-free diet, high in enzymes, also helps to dissolve atherosclerotic plaque and to clear arteries, so that the circulation of the blood improves, as does respiration."[7]

Despite their impressive medical credentials, both Gerson and Gonzalez have been vilified for their emphasis on coffee enemas in their healing protocols. When I asked Gonzalez why conventional medicine rejects coffee enemas, he replied, "Those in orthodox medicine can understand supplements, diet, and enzymes, but coffee enemas just make no sense to them. But when you're trying to repair a damaged body, when you're trying to get rid of pounds of tumor, you're going to have an enormous amount of toxic waste in your body. You need techniques to help get rid of it. Coffee enemas do that."

My Experience

I must admit that when Dr. Shamim told me I would need to do periodic four- to five-day cleansing juice fasts accompanied by coffee enemas, I was dismayed. Enemas! Puhleeze! That was bathroom talk. I certainly did not discuss bowel elimination and tried not to think about it. Although at times I struggled with constipation like millions of other Americans and especially so the year before I was diagnosed with cancer, I'd never had an enema in my life. But I felt so weak and rotten following surgery, with its plethora of drugs, that I knew I needed to do something to feel better. So I took Dr. Shamim's cancer-recovery protocol home and launched into my first cleansing juice fast.

I won't lie to you; it wasn't easy. For the first two days of the juice fast, all I could think about was food. Even with eight to ten glasses of freshly made carrot-apple and green veggie juice—about one an hour—I was ravenous. It wasn't until day three that I ceased to be hungry and felt greater energy. As for the coffee enemas, at first it didn't make sense that Shamim was telling me to give up caffeine while at the same time instructing me to insert it into my rectum. He assured me that caffeine taken orally does not have the same effect on the body as caffeine administered rectally and that coffee enemas would stimulate my liver and gall bladder to remove toxins, open bile ducts, and encourage increased peristaltic action.

Although I had never been to medical school and understood little about how the body works, I knew my liver needed help because my blood work showed that

I had high liver enzymes. As I told an overweight lawyer at dinner recently when he confessed that his doctor was concerned about *his* high liver enzymes, "You'd better love your liver. You may have two kidneys, but you have only one liver, and when your liver goes, your body goes." The man looked at me guiltily as he munched away on his high-fat dinner, little realizing all that fat was going to make his liver work harder that night. Not surprisingly, he was not amused by my comments. I understood. Until I was diagnosed with cancer, I knew nothing about the liver as the main organ of detoxification for disease, and I certainly had never heard about coffee enemas. In fact, had I not been terrified for my life, I would have tossed Shamim's instructions into the wastebasket.

What I can tell you is that coffee enemas have consistently made me feel better over the years; they have never made me feel worse. And I do believe they have helped me significantly in the recovery of my health. I understand what Gonzalez meant when he said that his patients who are ten and twenty years out from their diagnosis refuse to give up their program. "They tell me they are experiencing better health than they have ever experienced in their lives," he said. And the daily administration of those vilified coffee enemas is a primary cause.

I am convinced that one reason I am still a resident on this gorgeous planet is that I have worked hard to detoxify a sick body, and I stay with my program. As Dr. Shamim told me, "The detoxification of the liver is central if you're going to heal the body." He advocates that his cancer patients do two coffee enemas daily, morning and evening, when on a juice fast, and three or four a week after that.

How Coffee Enemas Work

According to Gerson and Walker, the coffee enema stimulates an enzyme system in the liver called *glutathione S-transferase* (GST), which assists in removing toxic products. When an individual administers a coffee enema and retains the fluid in the colon for twelve to fifteen minutes, the GST enzyme system increases in activity about 650 percent above normal, removing electrophiles, or free radicals. Gerson and Walker state that "the coffee enema removes ammonia-like products, toxic-bound nitrogen, protein derivatives, polyamines, amino acids," among other things.[8] This dumping of wastes through the colon keeps the body from being poisoned by its own waste products.

Gonzalez said, "When you take coffee rectally, caffeine stimulates certain nerves in the sacral region of the lower pelvis, and when those nerves are turned on by the caffeine, they feed back to the liver through the reflex arc and cause the liver to release toxins. It's neurological. You don't absorb a lot of caffeine. In fact, I had a patient who did a series of coffee enemas and had her blood drawn for caffeine, and it came back almost zero. You absorb some, and it immediately goes into the portal vein and into the liver, and the liver dumps it right back into the colon. So you get very little systemic absorption of caffeine...minuscule amounts."

What is happening is that the cholerectics in the coffee increase the flow of toxins from the gall bladder, the liver's "partner organ," and this aids liver detoxification. *An Alternative Medicine Definitive Guide to Cancer* states that "the coffee enema is among the only pharmaceutically effective choleretic noted in the medical literature that can be safely used many times daily without toxic effects."[9]

WHAT ABOUT COFFEE ENEMAS IF YOU'VE HAD CHEMOTHERAPY?

If you are on chemotherapy, should you self-administer coffee enemas? Charlotte Gerson and Dr. Morton Walker urge great caution in detoxifying the body during and after chemotherapy. They write, "Pursuing the full, unmodified Gerson protocol for any patient who has undergone chemotherapy, regardless of the time elapsed since the last treatment, can be extremely dangerous."[10] They advocate that those who have taken chemo follow a modified Gerson Therapy, reducing the juice intake and undergoing fewer coffee enemas daily. Specifically they suggest that patients treated with chemo take a thirty-two-ounce enema two or three times a day and that some may wish to reduce the enema's strength by mixing sixteen ounces of chamomile tea with sixteen ounces of coffee. Gerson and Walker state that "care must be taken not to overstimulate the liver and cause extremely toxic side effects from elimination of the chemotherapy residues lodged within the body."[11]

To better understand how to detox a body undergoing chemo, I turned to Dr. Block, a conventionally trained doctor who administers fractionated chemo and still believes in detoxification. Block told me, "We have found enormous value in providing detoxification in between cycles of chemotherapy and following chemotherapy and radiation. Enough scientific understanding now exists to allow for meaningful ways to eliminate burdensome toxic metabolites."

Then Dr. Block launched into a discussion of how the liver works in dealing with chemicals. He said, "The liver has the ability to break down chemicals, such as chemotherapy drugs (referred to as phase 1 detox), and to flush out metabolic by-products (referred to as phase 2 detox). The problem is overdoing the first step—the breakdown process—without increasing the elimination phase. Such imbalance can lead to drug interactions, causing increases in toxicity and interference in drug activity."

Block believes that clearing metabolic by-products too quickly reduces drug-influenced activity. "However, leaving drug residue behind can lead to treatment interference or resistance," he said. "This can be a real problem for patients undergoing multiple rounds of chemotherapy." So, according to Block, "Getting the dosing and timing of chemotherapy and detox right is clinically important."

To this end, Block recommends introducing glucosinolates from the *Brassica* vegetable group (broccoli, Brussels sprouts, cauliflower) and the *Allium* group (garlic and onions) along with high-fiber whole grains to encourage regular detoxification through the bowel. In addition, he recommends a milder detox when going through chemo (supplements, detox food, salt baths) and a more aggressive detox once chemo and radiation have been completed (infrared saunas, stronger salt baths, stronger nutritional and herbal regimens).

If you are struggling to regain your health after cancer, you need to find a physician who will work with you to detoxify your body—by using coffee enemas if you haven't taken chemo or by using the other forms of detox, as Dr. Block suggests, if you have undergone chemo. I was grateful that I had Dr. Shamim to work with me in detoxifying my body, and I knew I could call him if anything went wrong. I suggest you find the same medical support in the important task of helping your body rid itself of toxins.

Candidly, it hasn't been easy to talk about private, personal habits in print—not for this Southern woman. Initially I didn't plan even to mention coffee enemas. Gutless, I guess. But Dr. Shamim admonished me. "Dr. Hunter," he said, in his slow, deliberate voice, "detoxification is as important in the healing process as good nutrition. You must tell your readers how to detox their bodies so they can begin to reclaim their health." He's right. I couldn't in good conscience leave this subject out even though conventional medicine has a hard time with this.

Nor can I resist telling you that a friend once embarrassed me in a restaurant by saying to the waitress, "She doesn't *drink* coffee; she just *takes* it at the other end." The waitress was dumbfounded, and I was mortified. But my friend, who has diabetes, called yesterday, asking for instructions on detoxification, specifically on the once vilified coffee enema. Did I feel vindicated? You bet. Will I help her? Of course. Will I tease her? Absolutely.

❖   How to Make and Take Your Coffee Brew   ❖

Are you convinced to try a coffee enema to help your liver function better and to remove toxic material from your body? You don't have to have cancer to do this; in fact, at some of the most expensive European health spas, enemas are standard fare when a person is juice fasting. And even if you are not fasting but are flooding your body with better nutrition, including vegetable juice, you may wish to use coffee enemas as part of a cancer prevention program, as Dr. Nicholas Gonzalez and Charlotte Gerson do. If you have cancer and are *not* taking chemo, you may find coffee enemas helpful. Regardless of your reason, here's how to make and take the coffee brew.

First, you need to purchase organic, caffeinated coffee. Never use instant or decaffeinated. Put a quart of distilled water into a stainless steel pot, and drop three tablespoons of drip coffee grounds into the water. Boil the solution for three minutes uncovered and then cover the pot and simmer the contents for an additional fifteen minutes. Strain the coffee into a Pyrex glass bowl and add enough distilled water to fill a quart container. Allow the water to cool to body temperature. Believe me, you do *not* want a hot coffee enema! Pour a pint of the liquid into your enema bag, and lubricate the enema tip with healing vitamin E oil, never Vaseline. I pierce a vitamin E capsule, and apply the contents to the tip. Are you ready? Now the fun begins.

Place a towel on your bathroom floor, and hang the enema bag in your tub or shower stall about twelve to twenty-four inches above your head. Make sure you close the valve on the tubing *before* you hang the enema bag, or the coffee will shoot all over your tub or shower stall, and you'll have a mess. (Listen to the voice of experience.) Lie on your left side on the towel, gently insert the lubricated tip into your rectum, and slowly allow the coffee to flow into your colon. If you feel full, close the clamp, and wait a few minutes. Then open the clamp and try again.

When you have emptied the bag, lie on your left side in the fetal position, and try to retain the fluid for twelve to fifteen minutes. Sometimes you may not be able to retain the fluid this long, but on other occasions this won't be a problem. Evacuate the fluid, and even if nothing comes out immediately, it usually will within a few minutes. When you have finished, rinse out the enema bag, and store the tip in a glass container filled with water and bleach.

There you have it—all you never knew you needed to know about coffee enemas.

One of my friends who has experienced recurrent thyroid cancer suggested I put this information in the back of the book under the heading "Desperate Measures for Desperate People." Even though I did feel desperate five years ago, I don't view the use of coffee enemas as gross or shameful or dangerous or desperate. To the contrary, I have found this detoxifying tool a tremendous aid in my pursuit of health: a gift to a very sick body that longed to be well.

Nurturing Ourselves—
Selfish or Self-Preservation?

Learning to relax deliberately is the absolute bedrock technique for healing through the mind.
ALASTAIR CUNNINGHAM

It's never too late—in fiction or in life—to revise.
NANCY THAYER

People ought to know that nothing is more remarkable about the human body than its recuperative drive, given a modicum of respect.
NORMAN COUSINS

Julia and I stood together at a summer wedding reception, introducing ourselves as she munched cake and I, raw vegetables. Lost in the pleasantries of conversation, I was surprised when she blurted out, "I have a rare and aggressive form of breast cancer and have just started chemotherapy." As we talked, Julia told me her story. "In the past three years I have worked full time as a Realtor and have nursed three relatives who eventually died. My mother was the first, and she died two years ago."

I listened and then said, "Well, Julia, that must have been enormously stressful—all that caretaking and all those losses." I added, "Now it's time to take care of yourself."

As I left the reception that day, I was aware of a recurring theme in the cancer literature: Many of us who develop cancer take better care of others than we do of ourselves. Spouses, children, aging parents, work, church, community obligations, sick relatives—all tend to come first, before our own legitimate needs for good nutrition, exercise, relaxation, or even adequate sleep. We lurch from crisis to crisis, harried and stressed. Like Julia, we don't ask for help in caring for others but too often do it all ourselves. We run from a business meeting to soccer practice to the grocery store and squeeze in housework after everyone has gone to bed. We can't remember not being tired. And the result? We give until it hurts, and we get worn down in the process. We have cared too little for ourselves. One man I met at a Fourth of July cookout told me he was "profoundly tired" before he was diagnosed with non-Hodgkin's lymphoma, but he didn't stop driving himself even after learning of his disease.

If we are to get well, we must change this debilitating cycle and set aside time each day to bolster our immune system, not only with life-giving foods and supplements but with exercise, time in nature, and time to pray and reflect on our lives. We must listen to our hearts and feed our souls. Daily.

This is not selfishness; it's self-preservation.

WOMEN FIND SELF-CARE HARDER

Men may find it hard to take care of themselves, but many women find it even harder because we spend so much of our adult lives sacrificially caring for others. At a recent Duke University conference on women's health, Alice Domar, Ph.D., director of the Mind-Body Center for Women's Health at Boston IVF, Beth Israel Deaconess Medical Center, Harvard Medical School, said, "The stress level for women in this culture is the same as for soldiers." According to Domar, women have consistently reported more stress than men over the past fifteen years. Why? Researchers have found that women have more relationships and responsibilities in their lives than men. "Men worry about three things on average each day," said Domar, "while women worry about twelve." She suggests that women's health ultimately suffers from not only greater responsibilities but also a Martha Stewart–style quest for perfection, the challenges of balancing work and family, weight and self-esteem issues, and an inability to nurture ourselves.

"Until recently older women took care of younger women. No longer," said

Domar. "While there's still great social pressure for women to take care of others, no one takes care of us." Domar cited research that shows women believe that self-nurturance is basically a good thing, yet they rarely take good care of themselves. "Self-nurture is hard for women to do because we think it is selfish. We would never put ourselves at the top of any list of people to nurture; it's hard to get us even to put ourselves *on* the list."[1]

Yet we must learn to give ourselves the same empathy and wise care that we give our intimate friends, our families, or our coworkers. This is true if we want to *prevent* cancer; it is nonnegotiable once we discover we *have* cancer. For men, it may require making hard decisions about jobs and family lifestyles to decrease stress. It may mean cutting hours, changing careers, or taking a sabbatical to regain health. It may also require enlisting the wife's support in changing the family's eating habits. For women, it will probably require taking the lead with food preparation and juicing and booking appointments for nutritional counseling. For anyone struggling with cancer, now is the time to ask for help from the rest of the family. Those who are well can buy the organic groceries, prepare meals, and make juice so that those who are ill can concentrate on getting well.

Perhaps you don't know how to begin taking better care of yourself. Since we nurture ourselves in adulthood as we were nurtured as children, those of you whose parents met your physical and emotional needs promptly and consistently will take good care of yourselves in adulthood. However, if you were neglected or abused, you may neglect yourself and focus exclusively on others' needs. It's time to break the pattern. If you have cancer, you must. How to start? Ask yourself: What gives me joy?

PURSUE THE JOY

At the Duke conference, Dr. Domar gave all who attended her workshop two blank sheets of paper. Then she told the attendees, "Draw a circle, and divide your day into segments based on how you spend your time." So I dutifully made my pie chart. Then she paired us off and told us to take turns at quickly putting down the twenty-five things that gave us joy. Finally she asked, "Now how many of the things that bring you joy are part of your daily life?" No one present engaged in more than four of their joyful activities daily.[2] I had three.

It's your turn now. How do you spend your days? Do you go for the joy? If not, what changes can you make to inject more happiness into your daily life? Whether it is stopping by your favorite organic bakery for an occasional whole wheat or spelt muffin, taking an exercise or art class, spending time on a hobby, having lunch with a friend, or doing whatever else you love, your happy activities not only improve your outlook but bolster your immune system as well.

Annie, who had struggled for ten years with undiagnosed adrenal burnout, found that getting a pet brought her an unexpected level of joy. "I always wanted a dog," she said, "but had talked myself out of it. I traveled too much. My apartment was too small. Finally I decided to get a wheaten terrier, and I've been amazed at how happy it has made me. This little creature really loves me, and I enjoy taking care of her. I don't begrudge her all the walks, and I love playing with her, because it makes her so happy."

Pets. Painting. Golf. Grandchildren. Hiking. What would you add to this list for your daily life? For some, time spent outdoors, enjoying the natural world, is a newfound source of joy and healing.

THE HEALING POWER OF NATURE

"Fear blocks healing. You can't heal if you're terrified. The first thing you've got to do is get to a place of peace."[3] So said Thomas Day Oates Jr., a twenty-something insurance salesman who lived in a state of overwhelming stress. But his body couldn't take the constant drivenness, and it began to fall apart. First, with a "flu" that refused to go away. Next with draining, unrelenting fatigue. Then Oates started to lose his hair. As it turned out, he didn't have cancer but rather chronic fatigue, which explained why he had energy for only fifteen minutes a day.

The first thing Oates did was let go of his dreams of having a family and making lots of money. Next he released the past with its regrets, realizing that regrets sapped his energy and kept him locked in the past. Then as he became more aware of nature and watched the seasons change, Oates became deeply peaceful.

Soon "his external world of struggle was replaced with a rich internal world of exploration and learning."[4] As he regained his strength, Oates ventured into his backyard with a camera in hand. A year later he felt well enough to take photography classes and eventually film classes. Having discovered the healing power of nature, Oates decided to make a video to help hospital patients find the peace he had discovered. His work, *Pacific Light,* captures sunsets and sunlight along the Oregon and California coasts, highlighting the colors of the ocean while incorporating soothing music, and is now used in a hundred hospitals, including the Mayo Clinic. "The video…has been used to improve immune function, as well as to lower blood pressure and heart rates, to calm overwhelming anxiety and panic attacks, to relieve pain, headaches and stress, to end insomnia and to increase one's overall state of well-being."[5]

Out of one man's illness and the death of his dreams came a tool to help others discover, as he had, the soothing, healing power of nature. Nature not only beckoned Oates as he lay bedridden, but it nurtured his spirit and promoted his physical healing. Nature can have a healing effect on those of us recovering from cancer as well; in fact, during these years of reading about "remarkable recoveries" from cancer, I have found that most survivors included daily time in nature in their self-devised healing protocols.

Inge Sundstrom, for example, discovered in 1991 that she had shadows on her lungs. After a routine chest x-ray, "out came these pictures filled with dozens of white spots that made my lungs look like a star map," Inge told Caryle Hirshberg and Marc Ian Barasch, authors of *Remarkable Recovery.*[6] When her oncologist told her she had six months to live, Inge was enraged, then despaired. But as she lay in the hospital, she experienced a triumph of the human spirit and wrote in her diary: "No, we are not supposed to die as the doctors say. I refuse to sit in death's waiting room, refuse to prepare for my own cremation. I am not one of the people the statistics spoke of. Even if 999,999 die, I am the one that beats the odds, the one in a million."[7]

Remembering that her hardy parents, who were self-reliant homesteaders in Saskatchewan, believed that you had to be your own doctor, Inge began to take charge of her recovery. One key aspect of reclaiming her health was her determination to be outside every day. Whether she took a walk or rode her children's sled down the hill behind her home or walked three miles down Wisconsin back roads, across fields and farmland, singing loudly "The Happy Wanderer" or "Beautiful May, Welcome," she had to exercise her lungs. Outside.

Because of this and other life-enhancing choices—stress reduction, relaxation, improved nutrition, painting, dancing, an optimistic attitude, a desire to see age ninety, and the love of her family—Inge's tumors began to melt away. Her physician said, "It appears she doesn't have any active tumor. There are still a few small areas on her CAT scan, but my assumption is at this point these are all scar tissue."[8]

Who can say what ultimately healed Inge? All of the positive actions probably had a synergistic effect, but I especially love the image of this resilient woman trekking through the fields, in springtime and in snow, singing at the top of her lungs.

Go to the Sea

Shortly after I became ill, I felt compelled to start taking better care of myself, but it came to a head one day at work soon after my mastectomy. I had seen clients for several hours that day and was listening to a woman rage against her husband when I realized I was done. *Finished.* I couldn't take care of others anymore. Cancer had given me a new and compelling priority: me. If I were going to have a remote chance of beating this disease, I had to take care of myself.

Within weeks I had resigned from my job. I had no plan, but an inner voice said, "Go to the sea." So my husband and I packed some books, some casual clothes, my Champion juicer, and a cooler full of organic vegetables and headed for the ocean—the first of what would be three pilgrimages to the East Coast that year—just to walk along the shore and feel the waves lap at our feet and the wind caress our faces.

As I gazed at the ocean and beyond to the horizon, my terrible fear of cancer and death, which had washed over me like acid for months, slowly began to abate. In its place came a sense of peace. It would come and go, but it stayed longer each time, giving me hope. Walking alongside the ocean that first year, I realized that the God who had established the tides and placed eternity in my heart could most certainly take care of my sickened and depleted body and spirit. He was the doctor; I was the patient. As I sat on the beach alone just listening to the repetitive slap of the waves against the sand, I felt my heart rate, pulse, and breathing slow down. I relaxed for the first time in months, maybe years.

I remembered reading years earlier about a woman with breast cancer who had been told by a cancer expert that sometimes a change of scene promoted recovery.

Following the doctor's advice, she and her husband took a leave of absence from their jobs in the Midwest, packed their belongings, closed their home, and moved their family to the California coast. They took up temporary residence in a small weathered house by the water where the ocean, sea gulls, sandpipers, hermit crabs, walks along the beach, and star gazing became parts of their daily life. At the end of six months, nature had worked its alchemy, and this woman was cancer free.

Why do we hike in the woods, camp under the stars, go whitewater rafting, sail across sun-dappled lakes? We are drawn to nature and the outdoors for the relaxation of our bodies and the replenishment of our souls. The air, the bird calls, the smells of damp woods in fall, and the beauty of wildflowers in spring—all speak to the deepest part of our being. As I have gone to the sea or hiked in the Smoky Mountains or witnessed the mists rising on the mountains from my bedroom window, something profound has happened to me. Not only have I developed a responsiveness to nature that simply wasn't there before, but I believe nature has elicited healing within me.

Nature. As the psalmist King David wrote thousands of years ago:

The heavens declare the glory of God;
    the skies proclaim the work of his hands.
Day after day they pour forth speech;
    night after night they display knowledge.
There is no speech or language
    where their voice is not heard. (Psalm 19:1-3)

As we think about surviving cancer, we need to spend time in nature, preferably daily. Let's consciously crunch the leaves in fall, feel the summer grass between our toes, pick raspberries or apples at a nearby farm, and *go to the sea*. No matter how landlocked we are, we owe it to ourselves to make a yearly pilgrimage to the sea. I have a fantasy, or a God-given dream, of some day running a place of healing, a holistic cancer center, where those newly diagnosed with cancer can come to learn about their illness and ways to reclaim health. A place where they can be nurtured, educated, empowered, and given hope. Where would I love for this center to be? By the sea.

Exercise for Life

"Only 17 percent of Americans exercise every day,"[9] and this sedentary lifestyle is certainly true of most who are diagnosed with cancer. Yet exercise is critical not only in preventing cancer but also in surviving it. According to Drs. W. John Diamond and W. Lee Cowden, "Physical activity helps move the lymph through its channels and thus aids detoxification."[10] When we walk regularly, we not only increase NK (natural killer) cell activity, but we eliminate toxins from fatty tissue and increase the oxygen supply to body tissues.

The latter is of paramount importance because cancer grows wildly in a low-oxygen environment. Two-time Nobel laureate Dr. Otto Warburg believed that the root cause of cancer was "life without oxygen or anaerobiosis."[11] He said, "All normal cells have an absolute requirement for oxygen, but cancer cells can live without oxygen—a rule *without any exceptions*."[12] Unlike normal cells, whose primary nutrient is oxygen, cancer cells thrive on glucose. Since cancer cells cannot exist in an oxygen-rich environment, we need to provide oxygen for our cells through regular exercise.[13] One study found that men who walked four hours a week were 35 percent less likely to die of cancer than their sedentary counterparts.[14]

Thus, a well-exercised body has a better chance of preventing cancer and, if cancer occurs, of controlling its growth. "Vigorous exercise raises the body's temperature and increases the production of pyrogen, a special substance that enhances the function of white blood cells,"[15] those cells critical for fighting infection. Also, anytime we move our bodies vigorously, we stimulate the lymphatic system, which not only removes toxins from the blood but also undergirds the body's immune system.[16]

There are other reasons to exercise regularly. According to Dr. Lorraine Day, a former orthopedic surgeon at San Francisco General Hospital and a breast-cancer survivor herself, exercise gives us a stronger heart and lungs, better digestion, better elimination, the energy to overcome stress, and lower blood pressure. Day recommends that we exercise outdoors because sunlight electrifies the air, creating negative ions. "Negatively charged air inhibits cancer growth," says Day. "Staying indoors all the time—in houses, cars, and buildings—makes us sick."[17] When we exercise outside, we are exposed to both positive and negative ions. So put on your walking shoes or get on your bike, and hit the road. We don't have to exercise for hours a day. In fact, when I had dinner with a former Duke University physiologist, he suggested I exercise thirty minutes a day, and in these years since my diagnosis, I have tried faithfully to do that. In warm weather, I increase that time to sixty minutes, or two walks a day.

Pumping Iron

In addition to aerobic exercise, strength training is important, especially as we age and face the possibility of osteoporosis. Lifting weights keeps our muscles strong, and strong muscles lead to strong bones. As reported in *Time* magazine, "Studies have shown that even ninety-year-olds develop greater confidence and are less likely to fall and injure themselves after strength training."[18]

I have been lifting weights for twenty years, and while I don't look like a bodybuilder, lifting weights makes me feel stronger as I age rather than weaker. Five mornings a week I work out at the Asheville YMCA (yes, it's coed), where movie star Andie McDowell exercises occasionally. I love the hustle and bustle, the friendliness, being greeted by name, and the fact that I am often among seventy- and eighty-year-olds pumping iron. One woman who works out with weights three times a week told me she is a young, buff, eighty-three-year-old.

Recently I read about Jan Todd, a forty-seven-year-old history professor at the University of Texas, who puts my modest weightlifting efforts to shame, and challenges me to cease being a dilettante and become more serious about strength training. In the seventies Jan became the first woman in history to lift a combined total of a thousand pounds in three classic powerlifting events—the dead lift, the squat, and the bench press.[19] In 1982 she was inducted into the Powerlifting Hall of Fame and became the only woman ever to lift Scotland's famous Dinnie Stones, which weigh a total of 780 pounds. Pretty amazing, right?

But in 1989 this strong woman discovered she had ovarian cancer, and during her treatment she became so weak she couldn't lift a ten-pound dumbbell. Her doctor grimly said she had less than a 25 percent chance of survival, to which her husband, Terry, responded, "But when have you not been in the top 25 percent of anything you've tried?"[20] So Jan "directed the perseverance she'd learned in all those years of strength training to beating back cancer and the fear that comes with such a diagnosis." Jan told her story in *Health* magazine in 1999, and she was, by anyone's standard, a long-term cancer survivor.

Stretch and Exercise

As you plan your exercise program, consider adding two or three "stretch and exercise" classes weekly. When we move into young middle age and beyond, we become less flexible and almost frozen in some of our movements. So we need to find a rigorous stretch and exercise program. Just this morning I went to the YMCA and for an hour stretched muscles I didn't know I possessed. At the end of class we lay prone on our mats, listening to soothing music, and I almost went to sleep. Nothing makes me feel younger than stretching, squatting, doing push-ups, or bending forward from the waist and letting my folded arms hang like a rag doll's.

Regular exercise not only improves our mood, lifts depression, and pumps oxygen into our cells, creating an environment less conducive to cancer-cell proliferation, but it makes us look better as well. That is a tremendous plus, especially because cancer often forces us to deal with loss. Loss of health and a sense of invulnerability. Loss of body parts. Loss of life as we have known it. Fortunately, regular exercise helps us to feel stronger and regain our zest for life.

Race for Life

Several years ago I attended a North American Vegetarian Conference and met a trim woman in her sixties, clad in running shorts and T-shirt, who had an amazing story. After we chatted for a few minutes, she handed me her book, *A Race for Life,* and said, "Read this." Intrigued, I read and was inspired by the story of this woman's unusual recovery from cancer.

Ruth Heidrich was diagnosed with metastasized breast cancer in her midforties. After a double mastectomy, she entered an experimental treatment program with Dr. John McDougall that involved diet only. Even though Ruth's cancer had spread to her bones and one lung, she chose to follow a totally plant-based vegan diet instead of chemo and radiation. In addition to radical dietary changes, she decided to participate in the punishing Ironman Triathlon, which involves a 2.4-mile swim, 112-mile bike ride, and a 26.2-mile marathon.

In her book Ruth states that in the twenty years since her surgery, she has run six Ironman triathlons, over a hundred other triathlons, and sixty-six marathons. She has also been awarded seven hundred medals. In 1999 *Living Fit* magazine voted Ruth Heidrich one of the ten fittest women in America! Heidrich writes: "As I was training over the hundreds of hours with my rhythmical paddling, pedaling or plodding…I was giving myself suggestions about how I was getting stronger, healthier, and having my white blood cells kill cancer cells."[21] She continues, "For me, doing the Ironman was my way of taking control of my disease. Instead of doing nothing, or grasping at chemotherapy or radiation, I was being as active as I could possibly be. It's only a hypothesis at this point, but I feel that the feeling of loss of control when you are given the diagnosis of cancer is one of the deadliest aspects of this disease. And the only way I could counter that feeling and wrest control again was by setting my goal of doing an Ironman."[22]

BRING ON THE SUNLIGHT

Few of us will attempt an Ironman, but most of us can bike, in-line skate, or walk outdoors for forty to forty-five minutes each day. On sunny days we absorb health-promoting sunshine. Although dermatologists have told us for years to avoid sunlight because it gives us wrinkles, fries our skin, and causes skin cancer, many cancer-care experts feel that sunlight has healing properties. For example, Donald Yance, certified nutritionist, clinical master herbalist, and lay Franciscan, sees hundreds of cancer patients yearly in his clinic in Oregon, and he believes sunlight has countless benefits. It elevates mood, modifies our endocrine system, and, since it is the best source of vitamin D, protects against breast, colon, and ovarian cancer. Yance writes in *Herbal Medicine, Healing and Cancer:*

> It's best to expose yourself to moderate amounts of sunlight regularly; if you
> wear glasses, remove them occasionally and, without looking directly at the
> sun, let the beneficial light pass through the optic nerve to the pineal gland,
> which regulates several endocrine functions, such as biological rhythm syn-
> chronization and the sleep/wake cycle. We now know that melatonin, an
> immunostimulatory neurohormone and power-antioxidant, is secreted by
> the pineal gland.[23]

What about sun exposure and melanoma? Although the incidence of melanoma has risen sharply since the midseventies, Yance doesn't believe this increase can be accounted for simply by overexposure to sunlight. "Slightly more than half the cases of melanoma can be explained solely as sun-caused, but the conventional model does not explain the rest of them. I believe that the predominant theory suggesting that increased exposure to sunlight accounts for more incidences of melanoma is misleading and over-simplified."[24]

So what's to blame? Yance suggests that since there are higher rates of melanoma among indoor workers and those with higher socioeconomic status, other causes may be the increased consumption of trans fatty acids, exposure to artificial light and electromagnetic radiation, photosensitizing chemicals found in processed foods, drugs, and more than two drinks of alcohol per day. He suggests that to protect ourselves against melanoma, we need to eat a nutritious diet, drink green tea, and take vitamin E, lipoic acid, and zinc.[25] Lorraine Day concurs; she says that if we are properly nourished and are out in the sun at appropriate times, we are unlikely to get skin cancer.[26]

To enjoy the healing benefits of the sun without risking sun damage or melanoma, take the following precautions:

- Wear a visor or a hat.
- Avoid the sun between the hours of 11 A.M. and 2 P.M.
- Use an umbrella, hat, and T-shirt to protect yourself at the beach.
- Get yearly checkups with a dermatologist. If you have fair skin and lots of moles, get your moles mapped so your doctor can spot any evidence of change.
- Check your moles yourself frequently. If they grow, change color, or have asymmetrical edges, have a dermatologist check them.

Donald Yance does not recommend the wide use of sunscreens, stating that most sunscreens block only ultraviolet B (UVB) radiation and not ultraviolet A (UVA) radiation, which is 90 to 95 percent of the solar spectrum. While sunscreens may protect the skin from sunburn, this may encourage cancer if people stay out longer than they would otherwise.[27]

According to Yance, countries like Britain, France, Australia, and Switzerland that have greatly encouraged the use of sunscreens have witnessed a sharp rise in the incidence of and mortality from melanoma. He suggests that sunscreens also interfere with the skin's synthesis of vitamin D.[28] Consequently, Yance doesn't recommend using synthetic sunscreens except for one made by Aubrey that reduces oxidative damage to the skin and can be found in health-food stores.

SLEEP AND REST

My friend Susie, who has never had cancer and who, at age fifty-five, jogs three miles a day, often before dawn, tells me she can get by on about five hours of sleep nightly. While this seems to work for her, the value of adequate, sound sleep shouldn't be underestimated, especially for those who have cancer. According to Donald Yance, during deep sleep the detoxifying enzymes in our livers do their important work of excreting carcinogens and other waste products. "This is when the nervous system switches into its parasympathetic mode and the body changes priorities—from creating energy and digesting food to rebuilding and detoxifying."[29]

So how do we cooperate with our bodies and get the sleep and rest we need? Like President George W. Bush, we need to go to bed relatively early. He likes to retire around 9:30. This is an excellent idea, because medical research has found that the hours before midnight make the most difference in obtaining restorative sleep.

What robs us of sleep? Heavy, protein-laden meals eaten late in the evening, late-night television viewing, problems and worries, to name a few culprits. I have discovered that if I eat before seven in the evening and don't overeat, and go to bed before ten, having parked my worries outside the bedroom door, I am most likely to sleep deeply and not awaken during the night. On those nights I listen to a soothing CD that causes me to feel drowsy after about thirty minutes so that my head hits the pillow like a stone. But if I eat late, watch too much television, allow anxious thoughts to race through my mind, and fail to listen to my soothing CD, I'm up long after Letterman has said good night. Then I'm in the kitchen, foraging for a banana or oatmeal to produce the sleep-inducing tryptophan. On those nights I remind God that his Book says he gives sleep to those he loves, so what about me? Then he gently reminds me that I have to assume some responsibility for getting the sleep I need and that I have just engaged in bad prebedtime habits.

If you are a night owl who has trouble decompressing and relaxing, you may need to change your bedtime rituals. Consider the following:

- Establish regular "lights out" and waking times, and stick to this schedule, even on weekends.

- Adapt your social schedule so you can be home an hour before you go to bed. You can't expect to go at full speed all day and then suddenly stop and fall into a relaxing sleep.
- Dedicate the hour prior to bedtime to relaxation; stop all work, housework, television viewing, and anything else that makes it hard to decompress.
- Do some simple stretches to relax your muscles.
- Journal about your worries and stresses so that you don't rehearse your problems in your mind. One stress-alleviating technique that may work for you is to rate your worry by the likelihood of its occurring and track this information over time. You'll be amazed how many things you agonized over never materialized.
- Keep the bedroom at a cool 70 degrees; pile on more blankets if you get cold. Open the windows and make sure your room is dark. Darkness encourages melatonin production, which, in turn, encourages sleep.

You need your rest because your immune system recovers as you sleep. And when you are undergoing treatment and are weak or depleted, add restorative naps as you feel the need. Don't push yourself as you likely have for years; rather give in to your body's wisdom. Rest, rest, rest. And only as you feel better and stronger should you begin to gently implement your exercise program.

Music and the Spirit

Recently I was in a Southern Baptist church, and a woman from the famous Brooklyn Tabernacle Choir took the mike and belted out a song of praise to God. She had hardly begun when the audience bolted out of their seats to clap and sway along with her. When she finished, I brushed the tears from my cheeks, deeply moved.

Music is powerful in our lives. It calms us, excites us, thrills us, comforts us. It can lift us out of depression. It can heal our souls. It can turn panic into peace. Music even has the power to change our physiology.

When I interviewed Dr. Mitchell Gaynor at Cornell's Strang Clinic, he told me, "People hold on to stress, trauma, and anguish in their bodies, not just their psyches or their minds. So we do a lot of work with music therapy at the clinic." He continued, "Music helps us relax, and when we're able to relax, we are then able to see a lot of things about ourselves. In fact, sound that creates inner harmony allows us to look at our problems, stress, and fear without getting totally caught up in the fear itself."

According to Gaynor, music not only opens us up psychologically, but it affects us physiologically as well: "You can look at any system in the body and measure really profound increases in immune parameters that occur when you listen to music you enjoy."[30] His book *The Healing Power of Sound* states that music we love has the power to change us physiologically in the following ways:

- reduce anxiety, heart and respiratory rates
- lower blood pressure
- increase immune cell messengers, such as interleukin, and decrease cortisol, a stress hormone that depresses the immune system by 25 percent
- even boost endorphins, those natural opiates in the body, the "brain's natural painkillers"[31]

Gaynor recounts the story of the famous French physician Alfred Tomatis, who was called "the Einstein of sound" for his revolutionary research in the area of hearing and sound. One day Tomatis was summoned to a Benedictine monastery in the south of France because many of the monks were suffering from "a rare and undiagnosable illness." Their symptoms? Exhaustion and an inability to perform their daily tasks.

When he arrived, Tomatis found "seventy of the ninety monks slumping in their cells like wet dishrags." He soon discovered that these monks had previously chanted Gregorian chants for six to eight hours daily, but the new abbot had told them to desist and instead to engage in more useful pursuits.

Tomatis understood immediately that the chanting had motivated these monks, providing "fantastic energy food." It had also given a sense of meaning and purpose to their cloistered lives and had filled their minds and bodies with deeply religious music. He suggested that the monks resume their chanting, and within five months they had fully recovered and were able to resume their daily routine.[32]

So what kind of music promotes healing in our bodies? Research shows the best music to listen to is what we love, whether it's rock 'n' roll, classical, bluegrass, jazz, or country. I must admit that my taste in music might be considered lowbrow since I cut my teeth on the music of Appalachia rather than classical compositions. I also love British ballads and the music of the Brooklyn Tabernacle Choir.

Years ago I drove around Washington, listening to a male vocalist with the Brooklyn Tabernacle Choir sing on a CD, "I'm not afraid of the darkness." I sang along with him, substituting the word *cancer* for *darkness,* and my spirit soared. That song, which I played over and over again, lifted me in those early months when I felt cancer had me by the throat. It also buttressed my belief that nothing, not even this dread disease, could separate me from the love of God.

Recently I joined our church choir, and when I come home Sundays after singing in two services, I am in a great mood. Someone once said, "I don't sing because I'm happy. I'm happy because I sing."

Music as a healing agent for the soul has a long tradition. Psalm 33 says:

Sing joyfully to the LORD, you righteous;
    it is fitting for the upright to praise him.
Praise the LORD with the harp;
    make music to him on the ten-stringed lyre.
Sing to him a new song;
    play skillfully, and shout for joy. (verses 1-3)

Originally the psalms were meant to be sung, even shouted.[33] Ancient instruments included cymbals, tambourines, trumpets, rams' horns, harps, and lyres. Sometimes worshipers danced in tribute to their God. When he was old and "full of years," King David, who had danced before the Lord and written numerous heartfelt and emotional psalms, appointed four thousand people just to praise the Lord in the temple with musical instruments (1 Chronicles 23:5).

So listen to music you love every day, and whether you have a decent voice or not, sing.

THE RELAXATION RESPONSE

In 1975 Harvard cardiologist Herbert Benson wrote a *New York Times* bestseller titled *The Relaxation Response.* In his book he stated that stress contributes to major health problems, including hypertension, mild and moderate depression, cardiac arrhythmia, anxiety, insomnia, and headaches. As a result of his research, Dr. Benson found that a simple relaxation response could counter the negative effects of stress, reducing hypertension, alleviating depression and anxiety, healing duodenal ulcers, and eradicating all sorts of pain. What is involved in Benson's relaxation response? Two simple components:

1. Repeat a word or a phrase silently or aloud.
2. When your mind wanders, refuse to worry about your performance; just bring it back to the word or phrase you are concentrating on.[34]

This can sound strange to those of us who maintain a frenetic pace and struggle to make time to reflect and pray. But slowing down enough to grow quiet inside can be extremely effective in banishing mental and physical pain. If you are uncomfortable with this whole idea, you should know that Benson found that fully 80 percent of his patients chose prayers as the focus of their relaxation response. Dr. Benson suggests that Christians recite *"Kyrie eleison,"* "Lord have mercy," or a line from the Lord's Prayer such as, "Our Father who art in heaven."[35] One of Benson's heart patients who suffered from chest pains chose to say softly, "Jesus saves." As she engaged in the relaxation response ten to twenty minutes a day, her chest pain greatly abated.

One thing that makes the relaxation response so effective is you can use it in a variety of situations. You can meditate on a prayer while taking a walk, mowing a yard, or fixing dinner. You can focus on an aspect of God's beautiful creation, such as a tree with fall foliage, while eating on the deck. You can recite a line from a favorite hymn or psalm while jogging, driving, or cleaning the kitchen. It's a way of calming the mind and going quiet inside that provides great physiological benefits.

Some form of deep muscle relaxation is imperative if you are suffering from chronic or acute stress, which takes a heavy physiological toll on your body. And few circumstances in life are more stressful than getting a cancer diagnosis. Literally hundreds of thousands have used the relaxation response over the years to deal with disease and stress, and Benson's work serves as a foundation for many of the relaxation programs in integrative medicine today.

THE HEALING POWER OF PLAY

Finally, a wonderful way to nurture ourselves is to incorporate some form of play in our lives. Whenever I visit my grandson, I rediscover the therapeutic value of play. We have a game called Giant that I created and played with his mother when she was his age. The "giant" lies on the floor, lightly holding a ring or small object and pretending to be asleep. Then the "thief" comes, steals the object, and flees with squeals and obvious glee. Instantly the giant rouses himself and gives chase, chanting, "Fee, Fi, Fo, Fum, I smell the blood of an Englishman." Whenever I am the giant, Austin runs around the house, panting and yelling. If I pause to catch my breath, his little head peers around a doorframe, willing me to continue. At the end of the game, I am winded but happy. He is ecstatic.

Since I spend a lot of time at playgrounds with my grandchildren, I often join my grandson on a swing or follow him down the slide, hoping I can squeeze out the other end. And when I am not chasing Austin, I am playing with two-year-old Katie, a fast and daring walker. When she takes off, I follow, chanting, "I'm gonna get you" as she squeals with delight. Such simple games. Such deep pleasure. I'm sure a zillion endorphins are released in my brain as I experience "the grandmother's high," which can rival any jogger's. These sweet, sweet children take me to bliss and help me rediscover the joy of play that I lost years ago when life was too stressful and much too serious.

Several years ago my hometown newspaper, the *Asheville Citizen Times,* ran a story about a wife, nurse, homeschooling mom, and former Peace Corps worker in Micronesia named Caroline Magee, who was battling breast cancer. Although she worked in a hospital setting with doctors who practiced conventional medicine, Caroline and her husband, Ralph, began searching for information on alternative treatments. In time she started to eat a whole-foods diet—avoiding white flour, sugar, meat, and dairy products—and began taking herbs and supplements. She also saw a psychologist who helped her communicate her needs to family and friends more effectively and taught her to nurture herself. One day Caroline stumbled on an effective way to do this. She rediscovered play.

> When it was really hot, I went down to the river with my two sons, and the neighbor's dog jumped right in to cool off. Then my sons jumped in, too, and, as usual, I stayed off to the side, just watching. I felt the tension between being the adult parent and the child in me who just wanted to forget about obligations and just play.
>
> So I went into the river, and we all floated down the rapids together. It

was wonderful! I keep reminding myself that the past is gone, the future is uncertain. All we really have is this moment."[36]

All we really have is this moment. So true. But, by God's grace, we do have this golden, shimmering moment. And in this moment of loving and nurturing ourselves, we have an opportunity to ask: What would I love to do just now to capture the brilliance of this moment for all eternity? Shall I walk in the sunshine with a dear friend or listen to music I love or play with my dog? What will make me feel most alive and render the most pleasure? *Shall I play?*

You get to choose.

A Healing Place

I might have cancer, but cancer doesn't have me.
DANIELLE FORDHAM, Hippocrates guest

Curing is what physicians hope to do: eliminate disease and allow recovery. Healing is what patients must do for themselves. Healing is a deeply personal inner process of becoming whole again.
MICHAEL LERNER

I am sitting in a large room at the Hippocrates Health Institute in West Palm Beach, Florida, listening to my fellow guests introduce themselves. Outside there is a torrential downpour; inside thirty men and women gather. Some, like the lovely African American woman from the Caribbean, are obviously ill. Others, like the blonde with the high wattage smile and the Boston accent, appear healthy. As they begin to speak, however, it is apparent that these men and women have come to the number one health spa in the United States and the number one *cancer* health spa in the *world* in hopes of recovering their health.

Hippocrates was the first alternative medicine health center in America when it was founded in 1956 by Ann Wigmore, a Lithuanian with no formal education who cured her own colon cancer using natural remedies. From the inception of Hippocrates, people have come there with autoimmune diseases, Lyme disease, diabetes, and rheumatoid arthritis, among others. It has also been the place of last resort for many suffering from catastrophic cancers, the place where people have come when they have "failed" chemo, and x-rays have revealed new cancerous lesions. In fact, the majority of those who came to the original Hippocrates, housed in a mansion in the Boston area, had catastrophic cancers.

With the flavor of an AA meeting, we go around the room introducing our-selves and telling why we have come. "Hi, I'm Ann[1] from New Jersey. I have ovar-ian cancer." Next to Ann sits a petite young woman with cervical cancer. Then Bob, an executive from New York, says he has a rare and aggressive sarcoma that no one has ever survived. He tells the group he has come because a friend came four years ago after being told he had only days to live. Today this friend, who still fol-lows Hippocrates' program assiduously, is cancer free. It is apparent that Bob, who has just had surgery, hopes to replicate his friend's success. One perky brunette tells us she had surgery for an aggressive cancer growing behind her right eye. Now she wears a beige patch. Amid the heart-stopping tales of cancer and its recurrence, several women tell the group they have come for less serious health problems. A film producer has flown in from Los Angeles to stop smoking and lose weight. Finally, a couple, looking healthy and fit, tell us they have come to be part of Hip-pocrates' Health Education Program.

As I listen, I am struck by the sadness on the faces of many in the room, par-ticularly the beautiful young African American woman sitting across from me on the sofa. She has a dark half-moon circle under her left eye, and I later learn she has an aggressive brain tumor. She has already had rounds of chemo and radiation and has trouble walking and bathing herself. I discover that the attractive middle-aged woman with the somber face sitting next to her is her mother and that she has come to Hippocrates to care for her daughter.

After the introductions, the Hippocrates tour director, who also acts as the group facilitator, tells us, "About 50 to 60 percent of those who come to Hip-pocrates have cancer. Only about 15 percent come for prevention of disease. I came here because of recurrent prostate cancer about five years ago. Today there is no evidence of cancer in my body." He looks healthy to me as he stands there, sun-tanned and trim, clad in khaki Bermuda shorts.

THE HIPPOCRATES EXPERIENCE

During my weeklong stay at Hippocrates, my perception grew daily that this is indeed a healing place. Heather Mills, wife of Sir Paul McCartney of Beatles fame, came here when her body refused to heal after her leg was amputated below the knee. Coretta Scott King, widow of Martin Luther King Jr. and possibly Hippocrates' most famous American guest, has been here four times; her picture hangs in the bookstore near that of television star Jim Arness, another guest.

Brian Clement, along with his wife, Anna Maria, directs the institute and is quick to say he is not a healer. "I'm not here to heal people. I'm an educator and facilitator," he told me as we sat in his office on the fourth day of my stay. When people do get well, Brian believes it's because they have found the strength within themselves to go on, and they are willing to pursue radical lifestyle changes that promote healing. "There are no spontaneous remissions," said Brian. "People have to make permanent changes to live a healthy life.... They have to have courage, commitment, and the willingness to follow through, and when they've done their maximum with free will, they have to turn their healing over to God."

A former student of science who has studied all over the world, Brian is a great believer in free will. He feels people have to want to get well, and they have to choose life and health over illness. And if they are unwilling to assume personal responsibility for their health? "Then they won't survive," he says. "Sometimes they lack the strength to reinvent their lives, and we honor that."

When I ask why people get sick in the first place, he states, "When people are not living a full life with passion, they find ways to sabotage their life. Disease is the easy way. There's nobility associated with it. People will cry for you and worry about you. Other than those who are exposed to chemicals, pesticides, and radiation, etc., our improper lifestyle choices—negative thoughts, poor diet, and lack of exercise—bring us to the doors of death."

Brian says all this matter-of-factly and with the authority of one who has worked with thousands of cancer patients over more than three decades. As I sit in his office listening, I believe him. Since he is big on personal responsibility, he has little tolerance for whining. Outside his door a sign reads "Thou shalt not whine." He says, "I told one of the guests to leave my office after he insisted on whining. This man said to me, 'You mean I'm paying for your time, and you're asking me to leave?' I then told him to go outside and read the sign."

Although Brian and Anna Maria believe that the individual is responsible for taking charge of his or her own health, what so impressed me about this husband-wife team is that they clearly believe even those with advanced cancers can get well. This air of matter-of-factness about health and healing prevails at Hippocrates and is healing in itself. People who have been through routine but horrific cancer care in this country with all of its fear, painful procedures, death pronouncements, and discouragement finally arrive at subtropical Hippocrates, with its thirty acres of natural beauty, its Spanish-style architecture, its state-of-the-art equipment, and its warm, friendly staff who believe in the program, and their moods brighten.

As I observed the other guests, I saw them start to open up, become friendlier, lose some of their isolation and sadness. And that's when the real work begins. Hippocrates offers a life-change program. "You have to learn to change and like change. That's how you get well," Brian told me. "We're asking people to take giant steps. Coming here is like coming to Mars," he said with a laugh. "We help them; we nurture them; we give them the tools to change. Without tools and three weeks away from their old lives, the likelihood of change is small."

Hippocrates is a nurturing place, and the prevailing attitude among the staff is that it is indeed possible to "be well." This creates a positive atmosphere for guests who come to learn how to take better care of themselves. One of the most encouraging aspects of Hippocrates is that healing stories abound. Some are even posted on the bulletin board near the juice bar so visitors can read testimonials from those who have gone through the rigorous program and reclaimed their health.

I discovered in talking with the staff that each has a favorite story of healing. The receptionist, Carol, remembered "a man who came suffering with a virus he had contracted from eating seafood. The virus attacked his joints so that he could hardly walk through the door. When he first came, he lurched from wall to wall, table to table, in obvious pain. Yet six weeks later when he left, he literally skipped through the door."

Ron Diamond is another Hippocrates success story. He came to Hippocrates after he was told by his physicians at Sloan-Kettering that his particular type of cancer, bone marrow lymphoma, kills 100 percent of the time. Ron wrote about his experience at Hippocrates in the institute's newsletter:

> In 1990 I was diagnosed with terminal bone marrow cancer. Luckily my brother Harvey, who had written *Fit for Life*, answered my pleas for sympathy with, "Stop crying and get a grip on yourself. Take responsibility for your own life away from the so-called God-like doctors, and start to really learn about health."

I read a lot of books. I went on a forty-day fast and became a vegetarian. When I heard about a special center called Hippocrates, I called my brother and he highly recommended it. I was finally able to attend during January of 1992 for the three-week program. Those three weeks saved my life. Until then, I was, at best, groping around in the dark. My cancer left me while I was at Hippocrates, and I have not had a bad day since. My biggest problem is staying off my soapbox. I wish with all my heart I could enlighten the world about the truths that Hippocrates teaches.[2]

Ron Diamond, like so many I heard about while at Hippocrates, continues to enjoy good health. In fact, at the ten-year-mark he had a CAT scan and blood work done prior to a routine operation. The test results showed that he was totally cancer free.

Anyone who has experienced cancer longs to hear that others have survived this scary disease. I was frankly amazed at some of the results I witnessed during my one-week stay. After only six days on the program, which is designed for a three-week stay, the blonde from Boston, who had experienced acid reflux and stomach pain for over a year, told me her stomach didn't hurt anymore. Two other women on pain meds—one of them taking morphine for her oral cancer—were able to cut back or cease taking their medication altogether after just two or three days. Several spoke of greater energy, deeper sleep, increased hope that they could get well. This was powerful testimony considering that most of us felt either uncomfortable or downright miserable during our early days at Hippocrates.

The Program

Just what is the Hippocrates program that can, according to past guests' testimonials, cure fibromyalgia and arthritis and may even keep catastrophic cancers at bay? It is called a "life-change program" and offers a rapid transition to a healthier lifestyle by addressing mind, body, and, to a lesser degree, spirit. It consists of raw, organic meals served at lunch and dinner (there's no breakfast); nourishing, freshly made vegetable juices; weight and blood-pressure checkups; massages; exercise in the fitness center or the four oxygenated pools; colonics; and group and individual psychotherapy. In addition, on Wednesdays guests and staff participate in a juice fast to cleanse and detoxify their bodies.

Another key element of the Hippocrates program is the daily lectures at which guests learn how to care for their bodies. At one session Anna Maria, a tall, slender Swede and former nurse who has been consciously detoxing her body for thirty years, gave a lecture on "Lymph, Liver, Lungs, and Kidneys." She told us that our bodies would detox 60 percent of their waste during the first ten days at Hippocrates. She also said that in a period of seven years, all the cells of our bodies regenerate—good news for those of us with renegade cancer cells. She warned against sugar since "sugar in any form makes cancer cells grow." Hippocrates advocates a raw, living-foods diet that restores the body to an alkaline condition since disease grows when the body is too acidic. As she said, "A living-foods diet also aids digestion. This is enormously important since if you speed up digestion, you have more white blood cells to fight cancer."

Anna Maria pointed out that while our total cholesterol should be less than 150, on a living-foods diet it usually drops to 110-120. Too much cooked or processed food is anathema at Hippocrates, because the heavily processed foods most Americans eat create lots of uric acid, burdening the kidneys. Living food, on the other hand, greatly benefits the body by supplying oxygen to the red blood cells. We heard about a woman in her eighties who came to Hippocrates after having suffered from asthma for thirty years. "She had only 25 percent of lung capacity left," said Anna Maria, "but after fifteen weeks on the program, her lung capacity was up to 65 percent, and that's with no machines and no medications."

One of my favorite lectures was on the topic of enzymes and living food given by Brian in the airy hut alongside the pond. He instructed us in the benefits of eating live food as opposed to cooked, "dead" food since heating any food higher than 118 degrees destroys living enzymes. According to Brian, "Here at Hippocrates for many decades we have observed the reversal of disease in great part due to the enormous energy that enzymes bring to a diseased body. Thousands of successful health recoveries are in a great part due to consuming large amounts of enzymes through the use of living foods."

What, you may ask, are enzymes? Brian describes them as "positive charges that are at the heart of physiological healing." They raise cellular frequencies and thus create "greater immunological strength," causing an increase in T cells, NK cells, and white blood cells. Although we are born with a supply of enzymes, these must be continually replenished by living food. "The healing power of enzymes is absolute and proven," says Brian. "Almost every regulatory system in our body depends on enzymes and suffers by their depletion: coagulation, inflammation, wound healing, and tissue regeneration, to name a few." What we need to do, then, is eat enzyme-rich food to have greater stamina and better health.

What are the best sources of enzymes? At Hippocrates we learned that the number one source is sprouts. After that, fresh fruits and vegetables as well as sea and freshwater algae contain a plenitude of enzymes. Since this is so, we drank green drinks (celery, cucumber, and sunflower sprouts) morning and afternoon, downed two wheat juice drinks daily, and flooded our bodies with pure water soused with lemon juice in between.

Brian, who despite being in his fifties looks thirty-five (if you believe my informal female poll), advocates unequivocally that if we are well, we should eat a vegetarian diet of 80 percent raw, 20 percent cooked. Until then, he recommends people eat 100 percent raw fruits and vegetables for two years after diagnosis. The 80 percent raw, organic food should emphasize vegetables. The rest of the diet can be steamed and includes winter squashes, sweet potatoes (no white), and alkalizing grains such as amaranth, buckwheat, millet, quinoa, and teff.

What about protein for a populace used to high-protein weight-loss programs? Brian suggests that excess protein (anything above 5 percent) is the primary cause of degenerative disease. He points out that meat remains in the body for three days, is highly acidic, and drains the body's resources.

Because so many guests come with active cancers, sugar is also a no-no at Hippocrates, and therefore fruit is seldom served. Brian suggests that fruit be only 5-15 percent of the healthy diet, which translates to one or two pieces a day. When a person does eat fruit, it should always be eaten alone because it is digested more quickly than other food, and it should be eaten before noon.

I was familiar with this, having been introduced to the idea in Harvey and Marilyn Diamonds' *Fit for Life*. The Diamonds state that since fruit is mostly water and is virtually predigested, intestinal havoc results when we eat fruit with anything else. "Say you eat a sandwich and then you eat a piece of fruit—for example, a piece of melon. The piece of melon is ready to go straight through the stomach into the intestines, but it is prevented from doing so. In the interim, the whole meal rots and ferments and turns to acid. The very instant that fruit comes into contact with food in the stomach and digestive juices, the entire mass of food begins to spoil."[3] So eat your fruit alone.

The only sweetener Hippocrates allows is stevia, an herb that tastes sweeter than sugar but does not feed cancer cells or disrupt blood sugar.

Sounds pretty radical, right? It is a radical treatment for sick and sometimes dying people. Fortunately, most who come to Hippocrates know what they're getting into, and because they're so sick and may have already tried all that conventional medicine offers, they not only comply with the program but are eager to learn how to implement the Hippocrates diet once they're back home. To that end, during their stay, guests even learn how to grow wheatgrass and make their own wheatgrass juice.

SUBTROPICAL BOOT CAMP

When I interviewed Brian several days into my stay, I laughingly told him that the first days at Hippocrates were definitely a boot-camp experience. "You're right," he said, adding that he felt it would be almost impossible for someone to recover his health just by working with his health professional or physician out of an office. "We lock up people here and give them the tools to recover their health." What makes the first week feel like boot camp? To begin with, as the people listen to lectures on living foods, pure water, and colon health ("all disease begins in the colon"), they start the living foods program, replete with its twice daily green juice drinks and the magic elixir that constitutes the heart of the Hippocrates program—wheatgrass. In fact it was Hippocrates' founder, Ann Wigmore, who discovered the healing power of nutrient-dense wheatgrass.

Wheatgrass, one of the most nutritious foods on the planet, is loaded with calcium, phosphorus, iron, potassium, sodium, cobalt, and zinc. It is also filled with chlorophyll and amino acids and is a rich source of vitamins A, C, and B, especially B-17, a known tumor inhibitor. Wheatgrass is Hippocrates' "medicine." So powerful is wheatgrass that it causes the body to dump toxins rapidly, especially when you drink two wheatgrass drinks (two to three ounces each) daily.

During the first three days of my stay, I had a terrible headache and occasional nausea, which is common during the body's detoxification process. I also was quite tired and napped in the afternoons, something rare for me. In talking to other guests, I learned that headaches, fatigue, and nausea were par for the course during detox. A great sense of camaraderie soon developed as we congregated around the juice bar in the mornings to compare our symptoms. Fortunately, several guests were in their second or third weeks of the program, so they encouraged us to persevere and look forward to better health and greatly increased energy. And when we groused about the raw food, the veterans of the program proclaimed with evangelistic zeal, "Soldier on."

On the fourth day I felt great and was euphoric to learn I had lost four pounds. One overweight man lost thirty-five pounds in his three-week stay. But what gave me the greatest pleasure was seeing sadness give way to laughter and pleasure as the men and women started to rally. When I asked several of them what part of the program was making them feel better, invariably they replied, "The total program. All of it."

Caring for the Body

Although guests learn about the mind-body connection in illness, the institute is perhaps best at caring for the body. Not only did we guests begin to detox our bodies that first week with raw foods and juices, but we also began to experience soothing massages with exotic names, ranging from Thai to Swedish to Shiatsu—all of which aid in the detoxification process.

In addition, we got a crash course in how our blood contains the story of our physical and emotional health. As the results of the weekly standardized blood draw came back from the laboratory, each of us had a session with Anna Maria, who explained the results and then peered with us into a microscope at droplets of our blood.

Using equipment from American Biologics, Anna Maria performs what is called a live blood cell microscopy. Under the microscope, as one guest said, "Parasites swim, red blood cells are either single or clumped [single is better], and white blood cells munch along." "Guests can also see stress lines in their blood samples, indicating that trauma occurred five or ten years earlier," Anna Maria told me. "Our emotional history is recorded in our blood." Her words gave new meaning to the Old Testament phrase: "The life of a creature is in the blood" (Leviticus 17:11). She explained that the guests' blood profiles often change dramatically after three weeks of a live-food diet, juices, and detoxification. Anna Maria uses the results of the blood test and live cell microscopy to create an individualized program for each guest that includes dietary modifications, specific supplements, and electromagnetic work.

At dinner one night I found a young Korean woman peeling five garlic cloves—her daily dosage was fifteen—to help treat her iritis. Garlic, we learned, is a powerful antibiotic with a long history; in fact, bandages moistened with raw garlic juice were used to treat soldiers' wounds during World War I. To prevent garlic's burning sensation, this young woman had already drunk water from soaked flaxseeds so that the mucilage could coat her intestines and help "the medicine go down."

FASTING FOR HEALTH

A major facet of the Hippocrates program is the one-day-a-week juice fast to nourish and detox the body, thereby accelerating the healing process. Fasting has a long and stellar history and is part of the Judeo-Christian tradition, harking back to Moses and Jesus, who fasted and prayed for forty days. Fasting has been called "nature's surgery table," because when we fast, uric acid, lipids, residues from air pollution, pesticides, fungicides, and herbicides from the environment are released from the organs and bloodstream for elimination. The institute does not advocate a water fast, because 65-70 percent of Americans have trouble with blood sugar. Nor does it endorse long fasts, suggesting instead that faithfully fasting once a week adds up to fifty-two days a year. While fasting at Hippocrates, guests are not served sugar-rich vegetable juices, like carrot and beet, but rather juices made from wheatgrass or a mix of cucumbers, sprouts, and celery. In addition, garlic is added to some of the green drinks because of its curative powers.

Although I had done four- to five-day fasts during the previous five years and truly believe in the healing power of fasting, I didn't look forward to Wednesday, Hippocrates' fasting day, since I was already in the midst of an unpleasant "healing crisis" or detoxification. What all of us guests did look forward to, however, were the cold raw vegetable soups at dinner, signaling that the fast was over—for that week at least!

THE MIND-BODY CONNECTION

Although the heart of the Hippocrates program is its attention to the body, both Brian and Anna Maria recognize that diet alone can take an individual only so far. Since the emotional component of illness is huge, both believe that guests must deal with their emotional pain to heal. Anna Maria told me that "food is perhaps responsible for no more than 50 percent of the recovery of health. If we don't deal with our emotions, we won't survive." Then she said that if a woman with breast cancer came to talk to her and blamed her husband for her health troubles, she would not get well until she examined her responsibility for the state of her marriage. She said in all seriousness, "It takes two to tangle."

One way Hippocrates addresses the mind-body connection in illness is through group or individual psychotherapy with their gifted therapist, Andy Bernay-Roman, a forty-something, slender man with an easy, approachable air. During my stay I participated in a single group psychotherapy lesson led by Andy. To put us at ease, he threw balloons at us and had us bat them about in a game of indoor volleyball; then we lined up to give each other back rubs to the rhythm of soft jazz. I was fortunate enough to have a trained massage therapist give me my free back rub. When we were ready to begin, Andy told the group that he used to get angry with late arrivals, but he had learned how to get even. He gave each of us wadded up socks and said when a latecomer arrived, we should pretend we were meditating and then, on cue, pummel the unsuspecting victim, who by this time would be sitting with his eyes closed. The result? The "victim" invariably convulsed with laughter.

I watched as this talented therapist took a room full of people with serious illnesses and enormous life stressors and put all at ease. When the hard but exhilarating work of therapy began, I listened and observed body language as several talked about painful relationships, thwarted dreams, and moral dilemmas that were tearing them up and making them sitting ducks for serious illness. As always happens in group therapy, those who don't talk still gain new insights just by participating in the group process and watching the therapist interact with each person who is courageous enough to share. Of course, research shows that those who share derive the greatest benefit. It was an amazing two hours during which three people dealt with their painful life situations and expressed powerful emotions. I later talked to two participants who felt they had experienced life-changing breakthroughs as a result of the emotional and psychological work they had just done.

How Did They Rate?

If you think I'm positive about the program at Hippocrates, you're right. I saw people begin to change before my eyes, and I applaud the scientific rigor of much of the program. Also, approximately 75 percent of those who come to Hippocrates return to retool their diets or get reinspired. Since Hippocrates is relatively expensive, this says worlds about the effectiveness of the program.

What are its weaknesses? I felt there was insufficient emphasis on the spiritual aspects of healing. In all fairness, I was only there a week, and perhaps this received greater emphasis in weeks two and three. When I spoke to Brian, he told me that the Institute is actively working to enlarge its spiritual emphasis—while at the same time remaining nondenominational. People come with all kinds of faith experiences or lack thereof. Hippocrates does invite guests to go inward, and to this end, rooms have no televisions or radios. While the institute has no library or chapel, it does have a staff person who will discuss spiritual matters with guests. As a therapist, I believe that the spiritual aspects of illness and healing are of utmost importance and must be addressed. During my stay at Hippocrates, I met several other Christians. As one lady with breast cancer said, "God is in this place," and I agreed.

"I Can Fly, I Can Soar"

On my last day at Hippocrates as I was getting ready to leave, I walked over to the swimming pools to tell several people good-bye. I had formed friendships with men and women who, probably because of the seriousness of their illnesses and the uniqueness of the place, had spoken deeply and from the heart. As I got nearer, I saw that the lovely young African American woman, Danielle Fordham, who had been unable to bathe or dress herself six days earlier, was swimming in one of the ozynated pools while her mother, Sharon, stood nearby. When I asked Danielle how she felt, she said her energy level had gone "from zero to a hundred" and she felt much better. She had been having grand mal seizures before coming to

Hippocrates but hadn't had one since. She who had exuded such sadness the previous Sunday was now smiling and laughing.

As we talked, I shared with them some of what I had learned from the cancer experts about the power of belief in getting well. Sharon told me she and Danielle were Christians, and then she stood tall and proclaimed with all the authority of a preacher, "Abraham did not *stagger* at the promises of God. No matter what my daughter's MRI shows, we are going to believe she will get well. The Lord can do anything but fail. By his stripes we are healed."

I felt like saying, "Preach it, sister. Preach it." Then to my delight, Sharon asked her daughter to sing the song she had sung for the group the night before at "graduation." I had missed that event but had heard about the daughter's beautiful voice. With that, Danielle, who had been sitting in a chair, jumped up and with her rich, lyrical voice, honed during years of singing in church choirs, began to sing "I Believe I Can Fly."

After she finished singing, I hugged her. "Yes, you can," I said. "Yes, you can."

Later as my husband and I drove homeward, I thought, *That's the spirit of Hippocrates—the belief that one can get well. And that belief is at the heart of healing.*

MENDING
THE MIND

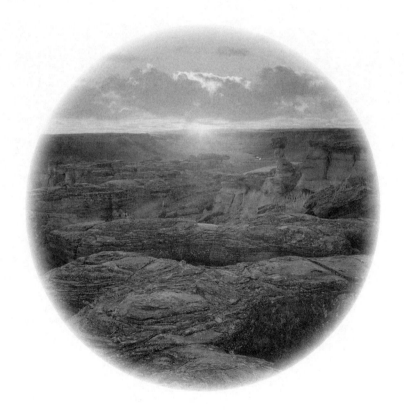

THE WILL TO LIVE

In the midst of winter, I finally learned that there was in me an invincible summer.

ALBERT CAMUS

I have cancer, but I don't want to fight it. I just want to go home.

A WOMAN WITH STOMACH CANCER

The man had been lying by the pool near the Sheep Gate for years. How long, no one knew for sure. What people did know was that he had been an invalid for thirty-eight years. For nearly four decades his life had been limited by his physical infirmity. His pain and disappointment with life must have been intense. Yet when Jesus came to the pool called Bethesda on that particular day, he did not command the man to get up. Instead, Jesus' first comment to the man was a question: "Do you want to get well?"[1]

Did he want to get well? Didn't Jesus know how long he had been lying by the pool, patiently waiting for the angel to stir the waters so he could be the first one into the pool and be healed? Surely this testified to his longing to be made whole and his ability to persevere.

Yet the man ignored Jesus' question. Instead, he complained, saying, "Sir, I have no one to help me into the pool when the water is stirred. While I am trying to get in, someone else goes down ahead of me."[2] *Pity me; I am helpless and powerless.* Then Jesus told him, "Get up! Pick up your mat and walk."[3] Instantly cured, the former paralytic obeyed and joyfully went his way, telling those who asked that Jesus had healed him.

Do You Want to Get Well?

If you are struggling with cancer just now, my question for you is, Do you want to get well? This may seem a stupid question—of course you do! After all, you have probably committed to a treatment regimen that may include months of difficult chemotherapy or radiation—all in the name of getting well. But the truth of the matter is, we can be compliant patients without ever addressing the core issue of whether we truly, deeply, want to get well. Yet our desire to get well is intimately tied to our will to live. If our bodies are to withstand daily environmental assaults and the bacteria that bombard us and to marshal a rigorous fight for life in the face of cancer, then we must possess a strong will to live. We must fight, every day, to survive cancer with God's help.

In 1964 Norman Cousins was afflicted with a life-threatening illness, a disease of his connective tissue. Told that he had one chance in five hundred—a .2 percent possibility—of full recovery, Cousins understood clearly that his will to live would be essential if he was to overcome his terrible odds. In *Anatomy of an Illness,* Cousins writes, "It seemed clear to me that if I was to be that one in five hundred I had better be something more than a passive observer."[4] Cousins continues, "Since I didn't accept the verdict, I wasn't trapped in the cycle of fear, depression and panic that frequently accompanies a supposedly incurable illness."[5]

Cousins' dire prognosis prompted drastic action: He moved himself out of the hospital ("I had a fast-growing conviction that a hospital is no place for a person who is seriously ill"[6]) and into a hotel room, where he was attended by an around-the-clock nurse. Fortunately, Cousins had a strong, collaborative partnership with his physician, who supported his desire to use megadoses of intravenous vitamin C to counter his collagen-wasting disease, as well as humor to engender positive emotions and reduce the need for pain medication. Watching *Candid Camera* films and old Marx Brothers movies, Cousins discovered that ten minutes of belly laughter a day acted as an anesthetic, giving him two hours of pain-free sleep. He says that he was "elated by the discovery that there is a physiologic basis for the ancient theory that laughter is good medicine."[7]

What does Cousins' remarkable recovery have to say to those of us struggling with cancer or those who want to prevent cancer? His recovery clearly illustrates the powerful health benefits of a strong will to live, active participation in one's own recovery, and a positive collaboration with a physician. According to Cousins, "I was fortunate…in having a doctor who believed that *my own will to live* would actually set the stage for progress; he encouraged me in everything I did for myself."[8]

In my conversations with long-term survivors, I have discovered that most share Cousins' indomitable spirit and strong will to live. Or if they did not initially, they realized the truth of their situation and made significant changes to jump-start their will to live after their diagnosis.

Quiet River of Despair

I only began to think seriously about my will to live when I read *Cancer As a Turning Point* by Dr. Lawrence LeShan. This was quite possibly the most important book I read early in my cancer journey, and it was certainly the most compelling.

LeShan says that feelings or emotions affect the immune system either positively or negatively, so when we have cancer, "the critical change needed to stimulate the immune system is an inner change."[9] In his work with hundreds of cancer patients, LeShan discovered that despair was often their basic orientation to life. He writes: "All the evidence from long-term individual psychotherapy with these people indicated that the emotional orientation of despair predated the cancer by many years. It had been the person's basic life feeling, their *Lebensgefuhl,* for most of their lives. There had been periods in each life when this background music was very loud and periods when it was quite low, *but it had always been there.*"[10] And their body's response to this ongoing emotional pain? The problem "was being resolved for them in a final, irrevocable getting rid of themselves."[11]

Why are cancer patients so prone to despair? LeShan found that people with cancer feared they could not be themselves. If they "sang their unique song" in life, then they felt certain they would be rejected and unbearably lonely. Or if they chose to be "pleasers," living for the wishes of others, inside they could not bear this total repudiation of self. The basic issue, according to LeShan, is that the cancer patient does not believe he can be who he truly is and be loved and accepted. Hence, the despair.[12]

MARIA'S STORY

LeShan recounts the story of Maria, a Brazilian pediatrician who left Rio de Janeiro and the work she loved to move to London so that her adolescent daughters could pursue acting and her husband, who hated his engineering job, could devote his time to writing poetry. Unable to find a job as a pediatrician, Maria worked as a pediatric oncologist. She hated both London and her work and missed Rio dreadfully. At age forty-eight she found a lump in her breast but for some inexplicable reason didn't seek medical help until a year later. Her diagnosis? Adenocarcinoma of the breast. Since the cancer had already metastasized throughout her body, Maria's prognosis was bleak.

When she met LeShan, who was in London giving a lecture series, Maria told him "she saw no possibility of work she would enjoy, of living where she would like to, or of a life that would make her glad and excited to get out of bed in the morning."[13] LeShan was struck by the depth of Maria's sadness and despair.

Because he was leaving London shortly and because he suspected Maria had not long to live, LeShan decided to be brutally honest. He told her he could see no reason for her to fight for her life. "By her actions, she was telling her body that it was always someone else's turn and never hers. Everyone else would be taken care of except her. Clearly she was telling herself that she was not worth fighting for."[14]

THE LOSS OF HOPE

How many of us had hope falter and nearly die in the years prior to illness? Whatever the reason, we lost our way and, more important, the belief that we would ever find it again. Clinical psychologist Ruth Bollentino, a protégé of LeShan who specializes in working with cancer patients, agrees that despair and hopelessness are concurrent streams running through the lives of her clients. "Not all the people I see are depressed, but often something has happened in their lives one to two years before the diagnosis that has left them feeling hopeless and despairing." She said that sometimes the despair resulted from the loss of a person, an identity, or a cause. She referred to LeShan's research that shows widows and the forcibly retired have a higher incidence of cancer than the general population.

Dr. Bollentino continued, "Sometimes it's the realization that a significant relationship is not going to improve. One woman who came to see me had three children and a terrible marriage. Her husband was a rageaholic who yelled and broke things. After being married to him for fifteen years, this woman suddenly realized one day that her marriage was *not* going to get better. She said she began to grow a tumor that day. Later she was diagnosed with metastasized lung cancer."[15]

Hope. How absolutely critical this emotion is for the very continuance of life. Proverbs 13:12 says, "Hope deferred makes the heart sick, but a longing fulfilled is a tree of life." While some humans can marshal hope and optimism while being tortured in POW camps, gasping for life in intensive care units, or growing up in dire poverty and abuse, others of us struggle to maintain a fragile hold on this powerful immune booster in more normal circumstances. Hope is, after all, desire coupled with the expectation of fulfillment, and the person who develops cancer has seen his desire too long unfulfilled. With the death of a dream come disappointment and despair. Early in the nineteenth century Sir James Paget wrote in his classic *Surgical Pathology:*

> The cases are so frequent in which deep anxiety, deferred hope and disappointment are quickly followed by the growth and increase of cancer, that we can hardly doubt that mental depression is a weighty additive to the influences favoring the development of the cancerous constitution.[16]

Why do those of us who develop cancer have such a tenuous hold on hope? I am convinced that feelings of hopefulness or hopelessness have their roots in early childhood. Our parental interactions and early experiences teach us whether life is "a gift to be enjoyed" or a "burden to be borne," as British psychiatrist John Bowlby said at an American Psychiatric Association meeting in Washington, D.C., in 1986. This "unconscious awareness" may go underground for years until something happens that reactivates these subterranean feelings. When I spoke with oncologist Dr. Keith Block at a cancer conference about the psychological aspects of cancer, he told me, "Some disruptive event often occurs several years before cancer is diagnosed, and this may lead the patient to revisit the emotional terrain of childhood. Some patients will respond to cancer with feelings of helplessness and hopelessness. Over many years of patient care, I've found this loss of hope among the most potent forces preventing a patient's ability to recover." On the other hand, in his study of long-term cancer survivors (ten patients with metastatic cancer who survived more than eight years), Block found that what these survivors had in common was they "were actively involved and fully committed to their healing and getting well."

But it is not always tangible loss that reactivates feelings of hopelessness. According to LeShan, "Sometimes the death of hope is brought about by the loss of the person's major way of relating and expressing himself or herself and the inability to find a meaningful substitute."[17] Cancer patients may be extremely successful in their professions yet not have found their lives fulfilling. "They could not find lasting zest and pleasure in their success and eventually had given up hope of ever finding it. The profound hopelessness was, in many of the people I saw, followed by the appearance of cancer," says LeShan. "Over and over again I found that the person I was working with reminded me of poet W. H. Auden's definition of cancer. He called it a 'foiled creative fire.'"[18]

FOILED CREATIVE FIRE

Auden's words resonated with me. Prior to cancer not only was I unable to find the right professional outlet, but my marriage was at an all-time low. While Don and I had experienced eight happy and intimate years at the beginning of our marriage, a second one for both of us, something happened when we moved to Washington, D.C., from New Jersey. After we packed up and moved south, our marriage followed suit. Don was stressed at work, we stopped doing many of the fun and nurturing activities that helped us celebrate our marriage, and I began a demanding, seven-year doctoral program. Unable to recover the early joy in our marriage, we poured ourselves into our work and the task of launching sometimes obstreperous adolescents. Exhausting! But we were conscious of the change, and in our quiet moments, both of us would have admitted we felt we had lost our best friend.

And then came cancer. One night several weeks after my diagnosis, a colleague called. Kathy and I had worked together at the mental health clinic, and though we were not close friends, I had told her some of the struggles in my life. This intuitive, wise woman told me, "Brenda, I know you've had a painful relationship with your mother and have been disappointed in love, but I urge you to choose life. I believe you might choose otherwise."

I might choose death instead of life? She had to be kidding. Agitated, I got off the phone and thought about her words. She had been bold enough to point out the quiet stream of despair running through my life, influencing my will to live. In so doing, she forced me to address the emotional truth about my life, something I had been avoiding. Why had I done so? Confronting the emotional truth about my life was exceedingly painful. Loss and despair had made repeated appearances in my life, starting when I was two and my father drowned. Immediately after this family tragedy my mother left me with my paternal grandparents and moved to a nearby town to find work, taking my baby sister, Sandy, with her. In effect, I lost both parents. When I had transferred my love, dependency needs, and loyalty to my grandparents, my mother reappeared after three years and traded children. Feeling that Sandy required the care a stay-at-home grandmother could provide, Mother took me home with her when I was five to fend for myself with a parade of baby-sitters.

When I tell various audiences my story of early losses and disrupted attachments, sometimes I hear gasps. They get it! The mothers in the audience understand just how painful and traumatizing those early parental separations and losses were for me. While Mother, herself a motherless child, was simply repeating the pattern of maternal separation she had experienced, my sister and I have paid dearly for her actions. Both of us have battled depression off and on throughout our lives.

After Kathy's call, I became honest with myself about the current state of my emotional life and acknowledged, yes, there were some feelings of despair. In naming the powerful emotion sabotaging my immune system—although I didn't know it—I took a first halting step in the healing of my emotions and my life.

During this time when I was reading everything I could find on the link between emotions and cancer, I spent a Sunday afternoon with my daughters, then twenty-eight and thirty years of age. I told them all I was learning about cancer and emotions and the will to live. "Mom, tell us your reasons for wanting to live, and I'll write them down," said Holly, picking up a yellow legal pad and pen. "What are they?"

I thought for a moment and could come up with only one—*one tiny but significant reason to live.* I named it, and Holly wrote it down. Then she quietly enumerated nineteen others and quickly filled the page. I understood what she was doing; she was trying to jump-start her mother's flagging hold on life.

I was startled by my response and horrified to think that my will to live, once a lively stream, had dwindled to a trickle. I didn't want to die, but did I really want to live? Ah, that was the question. And it is a question that many who struggle with cancer need to face head on. One woman who had lung cancer only began to get well after she confronted the fact that while she feared death, she wasn't that excited about living. If she wanted to beat cancer, she realized she had to whole-heartedly embrace her life.

To scramble to higher ground, I had to deal with all that was sapping my ener-gies and causing me emotional pain, and I needed to strengthen my belief that I could, with God's help, re-create a rewarding life that would give me abundant joy and zest. Earlier in my life I had experienced happy periods, so I knew I could be a happy woman.

The remedy? I had to address my unmet needs and resolve the pain in my key relationship: my marriage. I also had to manage or eliminate all the sources of chronic stress that zapped my immune system and gobbled up my energy. I knew I couldn't merely live for others—children, husband, even a gorgeous grand-child. Nor, in the final analysis, would any job be enough. As Studs Terkel said in *Working*, "Jobs are not big enough for people." Something needed to radically change inside—my self-perceptions, my feelings about the God of the universe and his love for me, my expectations—so that my will to live could once again be robust.

Although it would be a long time before I could honestly say I wanted to live simply because I loved life, and my life in particular, I felt comforted once I decided to fight for my life. An inner, seismic shift occurred. Determined to learn all I could about healing inside and out, I was no longer drifting. Instead I began swimming upstream as hard and fast as I could.

CHOOSING LIFE

In her book *Promoting a Fighting Spirit*, psychologist Dr. Linda Seligman, herself a long-term breast-cancer survivor, suggests there are four characteristic responses that individuals have to a cancer diagnosis:

1. The fighting spirit—These individuals accept their diagnosis, are opti-mistic, and seek resources to help them fight the disease.

2. Positive avoidance (denial)—These people reject the diagnosis or minimize its seriousness.

3. Fatalism (stoic acceptance)—While accepting their diagnosis, these individuals don't seek out information because they don't believe they have any personal power or efficacy. Their future is in the hands of others—God or their medical team.

4. Helpless/hopeless—These individuals feel "overwhelmed and consumed" by their disease.[19]

Which group is most likely to survive cancer? Dr. Seligman says that at the five- and ten-year marks those characterized by a fighting spirit "were significantly more likely to be alive and disease-free than those people whose responses had been characterized by fatalism or hopelessness. Interestingly, the group characterized by denial also had a relatively positive outcome."[20] But Seligman suggests that although they are spared the worry and discouragement that consumes the other groups, those who deny the seriousness of their disease do not experience the sense of control and empowerment that fighters do.

Dr. James Gordon, a psychiatrist who is the founder and director of the Center for Mind-Body Medicine in Washington, D.C., agrees that "people who feel hopeless and helpless do less well." He suggests further that "people who do better are the ones with a fighting spirit or those in total denial, who say, 'It's not going to bother me. Cancer, smancer, who cares.' All of us have seen people like that who outlive anybody's expectations."[21]

So what should you do if you currently feel helpless and hopeless? Dr. Gordon believes it's important to acknowledge how you feel and move on. "The goal is to move into the stage where the way you're coping with cancer makes you feel better and gives you some sense of mastery, engagement, and control." He added, "The key is to help people become more engaged in their own healing and not just be passive recipients of whatever approach they choose to follow. It's critical that people with cancer take an active role in their care and view the illness as more of a challenge and less of a catastrophe." Dr. Gordon then told me about an eighty-six-year-old woman with lung cancer with whom he is currently working. "She has decided to keep on trucking. In fact, she looks better now than she did many months before she was diagnosed with cancer."

What about you? How engaged are you in your recovery? Cancer asks: Is your life worth fighting for? Are you just existing, drifting through life, or do you bound out of bed in the morning eager to live the day? Are you willing to search for the medical help you need and make the necessary changes in lifestyle so that your body can possibly recover, or are you living for others while denying your own legitimate needs, too discouraged to believe they will ever be met? Can you imagine that you could retool your life and feel fully alive, or have you run out of dreams and can't envision being excited about life again? Now is the time for soul-searching and truth telling. Get a notebook and begin to journal about your will to live. On a scale of 0 to 10, how strong would you rate it? Do you believe you can, with God's help, live in a way that satisfies your deepest psychological, intellectual, and spiritual needs?

No matter how successful you are, don't be fooled by your workaholism, your career success, your myriad achievements. I have talked to some very successful people who told me they have never been close to anyone. They suffer intensely because of a lack of intimate, loving relationships. I have also talked to others who said they wanted to live for a husband, a child, or a grandchild. Usually these were women who banked everything, including their lives, on their relationships. The truth is, we cannot live for others or for success or for any achievement—anything external to ourselves except God. To strengthen our will to live, we must come to the point where we want to live because we cherish life itself, and our own life in particular.

How well I remember the day psychotherapist Dorothy (Didi) Firman, one of the directors of the Synthesis Center in Amherst, Massachusetts, asked me a paradoxical question: "Would you be willing to leave your husband, your children, your grandchild and move to another state for a time if your life depended on it?" Surprised, I nonetheless understood the question behind the question. I knew, and so did she, that this wasn't about leaving my family at all. Rather it was about making myself important enough to do whatever it took to heal. Didi could as easily have asked if I would leave the country to save my life.

I answered yes. By this time I had made the healing of my body and my life my number one priority, and I was strong enough emotionally to do whatever it took to get well. What about you? Do you love yourself enough to do whatever it takes to get well? I truly hope so.

We cannot live for achievement, causes, or human relationships—even those family relationships that are so important to us. Ultimately, we can only live for God and for the tasks he gives us to glorify him. He alone can supply the sense of meaning and purpose we long for as humans. Neuroscience has discovered that just as we are hardwired to connect as babies, we are hardwired to search for, and find, meaning and purpose in our lives. With God's help, we can not only discover why we were created in the first place, but we can embrace life with all of its challenges, pain, frustration, and joy after cancer. What happens when we give our bodies the unflinching message that we will do whatever it takes to fight for our lives? The immune system hears and responds. *Ah, it says, this is a life worth fighting for.*

THE POWER OF BELIEF

Do you believe you can survive cancer, even in the face of your particular death statistics and the naysayers? Dr. Bollentino told me that she refuses to work with individuals who do not believe they can get well. That does not mean she refuses to work with those who are terrified by their doctor's death statistics. "It makes me angry that I have to spend initial sessions undoing what their oncologists have told them," she said as we sat in her office in New York City. "I tell my patients, 'Nobody knows how long you will live.'" She told me that Larry LeShan used to ask his patients, "Does your doctor have a golden telephone that can ring up God?" Bollentino continued, "Usually I know someone with the same diagnosis who has survived, so I say, 'Why not you?'" Then she added, "Unfortunately, if someone believes he is going to die, he probably will."[22]

Belief is powerful. It shapes the course of our lives. It brings great happiness or floods us with feelings of terror and desperation about our capacity to get well. It's strategic that we examine our core beliefs about ourselves, our right to joy and happiness, our capacity to beat cancer. As I have interviewed the experts, I have posed one question to each of them: What do those who survive cancer have in common? When I interviewed Dr. Mitchell Gaynor at the Strang Cancer Institute, he said that many cancer survivors share two characteristics: "First, they believe they can get well, and, second, they are willing to change their lifestyle in beneficial ways to facilitate their healing."[23]

That sounds like a fighting spirit to me.

ONE IN A HUNDRED

Among cancer survivors, Lucius Morton stands out because of his strong will to live. In 1993 he was diagnosed with metastasized, stage 4 renal cell carcinoma. When Lucius and his wife, Suzanne, consulted with his urologist, the doctor told them, "Lucius has a tiger by the tail. There is no cure for this disease, and you, Lucius, have between eighteen and twenty-four months to live." Suzanne's reply? "Doctor, that's not good enough."

Within weeks Lucius had decided to travel to M.D. Anderson Hospital in Houston, Texas, because among the large cancer centers, this one had warmer March weather. "I like warm weather better than cold weather," drawled this Georgian, who had a kidney removed before he made the trip to Texas. The night before he flew to Houston he told his wife, "If I have a limited time to live, we're going to sell our stocks, go to Europe, and have the best time in our lives. We've never been to Europe, and we need to go and have fun." That same Friday night he and Suzanne entertained many of their friends, who came to offer support and to pray. The friends left at three in the morning even though Lucius and Suzanne had a plane to catch in just a few hours.

Touched by the love of his friends, Lucius didn't sleep at all that night, and by morning he was a changed man. He had resolved to live. He told his sleepy wife that instead of preparing to die, he was going to fight for his life, no matter what it took. "I made a conscious decision that I was going to live to see my grandchildren," said this man whose two daughters have yet to marry. With that attitude he and Suzanne flew to Houston, where he had "every test but a pap smear" in order to qualify for a particular chemotherapy protocol. Lucius told the doctor who interviewed him, "If there are a hundred people in this protocol and only one makes it, I intend to be that one. I will pray for, and feel sorry for, all the rest."

How's that for a fighting spirit! Among the fifty-two people in Lucius's study, one died from the treatment itself, and only four patients went into remission. Lucius stands tall among the four. According to Suzanne, Lucius was the first person with renal cell carcinoma that had metastasized to the bone (it usually metastasizes to the soft tissue) who had a 100 percent response to chemotherapy.

"I never thought I would die after that night," said Lucius. "I was never hopeless."

When Lucius reflects on what led up to his cancer, he admits that about two years before he became ill, he experienced severe loss. He lost his daughters, whom he had raised for eight years following his divorce, when they decided they wanted to live with their mother. At the same time, he and Suzanne broke off their seven-year relationship. "That was a horrible time," said Lucius. Fortunately, he and Suzanne married several months later but not before his body and immune system had registered these losses.

About two years after he and Suzanne married, Lucius discovered he had cancer. "Suzanne and I do well in pulling through adversity," said Lucius. She told me she loves his sense of humor, his ability to be scared and joke about it. "I love Lucius for his love of life, his morals, his standards, and the fact that his children came first when we were dating," she said.

Lucius ended our conversation by saying that others struggling with cancer often call him. "I can sometimes hear in their voices and in the words they say if they are going to make it or not. I tell them, don't worry about dying; that may increase your chance of dying. I also tell them I've always appreciated life; I've loved life. And I believe if you have a sense of humor, it will help you recover and get the most out of life." Wise words.

THE END OF MARIA'S STORY

Whatever happened to Maria, the Brazilian pediatrician who was filled with sadness and despair when she met Dr. LeShan? In their one conversation, LeShan challenged her to love herself and take action to enhance her will to live. That very night Maria gathered the family and told them it was her time now. She informed her husband that he would need to get a job to support his writing and her daughters that they would need to work part time to fund their acting lessons. Maria then quit her job in oncology and began a residency in pediatrics. Someday she hopes to move back to Brazil, but in the meantime she returns for a visit each summer. The result of Maria's life-embracing decisions? Four years later she was alive and well and doing the work she loved. Her body had gotten the message that she was worth fighting for.

What about you? Is your life worth fighting for, or will you passively accept the prognosis your doctor gives you? Have you been denying your deepest needs in order to please others or to meet someone else's expectations? Will you do whatever you need to do or go wherever you need to go to get well? *Will you choose life?*

And if you have never had cancer but realize that you have unresolved childhood wounds, or struggle with depression, or live for externals—job, relationships, causes, or possessions—are you willing to honestly assess the strength of your will to live?

Prevention is easier than repair. Always. And prevention means being honest about where we are in our lives and how much joy we experience on a daily basis. We need to consciously choose life. Today.

As Andie McDowell says in the L'Oreal commercial, "You're worth it." Yes! Who knows but that "the best is yet to be, the last of life, for which the first was made."[24]

CHRONIC STRESS
AND CANCER

Stress can wreak havoc on your metabolism, raise your blood pressure, burst your white blood cells,...ruin your sex life, and if that's not enough, possibly damage your brain.

ROBERT SAPOLSKY

Chronic, inescapable, or unpredictable stress appears to be the more significant causal factor in human diseases.

CANDACE PERT, HENRY DREHER, MICHAEL RUFF

Julie knows how it feels to have life spiral out of control. In February 1985 her husband, Jim, a local newscaster, was diagnosed with ALS (Lou Gehrig's disease), her mother was diagnosed with Alzheimer's, and she learned her adult daughter was addicted to drugs. "It was so hard to digest that Jim had this terrible disease and he was going to die, and my mother's mind was going at the same time so I couldn't talk to her about what was going on," Julie told me. "Then we found out that our adult daughter was taking amphetamines and lying about it.

"For the first time in my life, I felt completely overwhelmed. All these things were happening, and I felt really numb. I shut down emotionally. I felt if I cried, I would never stop. I didn't know where to begin a conversation about any of those things because it was so devastating." Julie continued, "We lived in a small community at the time, and Jim was well known. I was extremely frustrated with the way he was handling the news of his disease. It was almost total denial. He hoped that his doctor was wrong, so his attitude was let's not talk about it yet but just wait and see. I was fearful about my own future, then felt guilty for worrying about *my* future when my husband had this horrible disease.

"Now I'll throw in the kicker," she said. "I got a letter from a woman in a nearby state who claimed Jim had fathered her child, which turned out to be true. My husband had slept with her before he was diagnosed, and I thought, 'What terrible thing is going to happen next?' It was as if all the things I had taken for granted were being ripped away from me and I was falling into a bottomless pit."

By this time Jim had lost the use of his arms and was totally dependent on Julie. "I confronted him about the affair, and he admitted it. He said he felt ashamed. I was so hurt and angry that I threw away my wedding ring. I know this hurt him, but I felt my marriage had been deeply violated. After that I shut up about everything," said Julie. "I considered leaving him, but I realized I would need to live with myself when it was all over, and I knew I needed to be a positive role model for our four children. So I prayed, 'Dear Lord, I can't fix any of these things. I don't know why they're here or why my life is like this right now, but help me through this. I need grace, peace, and strength.'"

Julie's faith guided her decisions and enabled her to care for her husband with love and compassion over the next five years. Fortunately, Jim never lost his voice and was able to continue working until he died. But each day Julie brushed his teeth, helped him go to the bathroom, dressed him, fed him, got him ready for work, and protected his reputation. Although they told their children about the child Jim had fathered, no one else in Sausalito knew that their famous resident was anything but noble and upright. Over time Julie forgave Jim, and their last years together were rich, filled with happy times with friends and family.

The night Jim stopped breathing, Julie was unaware he had died. Although he was hooked to a ventilator, she usually slept with her hand on his chest to monitor his breathing, but that night she slept deeply. Early the next morning her son, who was living at home, woke her to tell her that Jim was gone. She told me that the hours after Jim's death were luminous; a soft, white light filtered though the bedroom window, filling the room with a sense of warmth and peace. In those early morning hours God's presence was very real to her.

Several years after Jim's death, Julie discovered she had breast cancer. I asked her if she felt the stress of Jim's illness coupled with her loss of faith in his fidelity had anything to do with her illness. She, like most women who get breast cancer, responded without hesitation, "Do I think my stress caused my illness? Yes, I do. I had so much stress for years, and I held a lot of stuff inside. I think that's what made me sick."

CHRONIC STRESS AND CANCER

Since I believed that years of chronic stress had factored into my health crisis, I was curious if other cancer survivors had also experienced chronic stress prior to their diagnosis. So I asked those I interviewed to tell me about their stress levels in the years before cancer. If they looked at me quizzically, I added, "You know, the kind of stress that refuses to go away but just sits there on your shoulder, confronting you daily so that over time it starts to feel normal." Invariably these men and women began to tell me about stresses they measured in terms of *years,* not months or days.

For some it was the stress of caring for a relative with a severe illness or the distress of having an adult child run amuck. For others, it was financial stress or a mind-numbing career that sapped their time and energy, making them feel helpless and hopeless. Some chronicled marital distress, ranging from divorce to the pressure of trying to blend two warring groups of children. What was key was the *chronicity* of the stress, the fact that they felt locked in stressful situations for years and could see no end to it.

For Larry Burkett, chairman of the board of Crown Financial Ministries (formerly known as Christian Financial Concepts) and popular radio host, certain events converged to produce several intensely stressful years before he was diagnosed with cancer. Larry, an open and engaging man who had published more than seventy books (totaling 11 million copies) about biblical financial principles, told me of the years leading up to his cancer diagnosis in 1995.

> We had moved our training center for the ministry to a site forty miles north of Atlanta, and it was virtually a disaster. I was traveling all the time; in fact, I traveled about fifty times a year at that point. Also, the ministry was audited by the Internal Revenue Service, and the auditor was determined to make my life as miserable as possible. We had many problems with the center and the staff. I went into overdrive. I became hyper. I walked and walked—sometimes fifteen to twenty miles a day. I couldn't stop walking. Moreover, I

didn't sleep well, and it was unusual for me to get more than a few hours sleep each night. It was a time of heavy, heavy stress. I could feel myself running down. I honestly believe the stress contributed to depressing my immune system and eventually to my being diagnosed with metastasized renal cell carcinoma.[1]

IMAGES OF ENTRAPMENT

Cancer survivors often use images of entrapment to describe how they felt in the years leading up to cancer.

Rachael, a survivor of lymphoma, had a high-stress job as a vice president of an imploding tech firm at the time she became ill. Struggling both to keep her volatile boss happy and to care for her sick mother, she told me, "I felt as though I were trapped in a room and rats were nibbling me to death."

Tom, who described himself as "haggard, stressed, and anxiety-ridden," watched his sick father deteriorate over a two-year period. As he and his wife struggled to provide the around-the-clock care his father needed, Tom said he felt as if he were chained to an out-of-control treadmill and couldn't get off.

Leona, a forty-seven-year-old director for a national public relations firm, told me that the two years before she was diagnosed with melanoma were intensely stressful. She had three young children—ages five, eight, and eleven—when her father died. He had had multiple sclerosis since Leona was five years old. "My mother, who had cared for him for twenty-five years, became suicidal and fearful. She kept a gun under her pillow, thinking someone would break into her house." During that time, Leona felt compelled to call her mom three times a day just to check on her. Also, Leona and her family moved from Colorado to New Jersey because her husband was having career problems, leaving behind all her supportive girlfriends. "It was a great loss since I was open with them and they with me, and we helped each other through all our struggles."

At the time Leona was diagnosed with melanoma, her husband, whom she describes as a good man, was suffering from undiagnosed bipolar disorder. Understandably, "there was a lot of anxiety at home." She added, "When you live with someone with bipolar disorder, and he's not on medication, you never know when you're going to fall through the ice. I tried to be perfect, not moody or demanding, just real, real helpful. My husband, who is mostly manic, would get very talkative and angry. I thought his moodiness was caused by my actions."

Now an eleven-year cancer survivor, Leona reflects on those years preceding cancer. "I felt like a beautiful bird locked in a cage. I was almost dying inside that cage because I didn't have a sense of freedom. It was as if the circumstances in my life were locking me up. But even in my worst moments, I believed that if that door would just open, I'd fly out and become a healthier person."

I remember telling Don just weeks before I found the lump that I felt as though I were in a jail cell and someone had thrown away the key. I was overwhelmed by book deadlines, caring for my sick mother, my heavy caseload of depressed patients, and the tensions in my marriage. In addition, my daughters were leaving home for college, and it was emotionally wrenching to think we would have no more after-school conversations or Saturday shopping expeditions. I felt powerless to change the things that were stressing me, and they preoccupied me daily. On top of this, Don retired unexpectedly, capitalizing on an early retirement buyout, and I lost my personal space at home, along with a fourth of our income. My life felt unmanageable.

UNDERSTANDING THE BODY'S RESPONSE TO STRESS

What happens when we begin to believe that this is the way life is supposed to be? What message does the body receive when chronic stress becomes the natural order of things?

Our bodies are marvelously equipped to handle acute, or short-term, stress. When an emergency arises, our bodies respond with "fight or flight," pumping out adrenaline and cortisol to enable us to combat the problem. But our nervous systems respond differently to chronic stress, according to the *Harvard Mental Health Letter*. Whereas our bodies respond to acute stress as a healthy challenge, chronic stress turns "the emergency response into a condition that persists when it no longer has any use."[2] This continuous state of inner emergency can have devastating physiological effects.

In his informative and engaging book *Why Zebras Don't Get Ulcers,* Robert M. Sapolsky, professor of biological sciences and neuroscience at Stanford University, writes about stress and its physiological effects. According to Sapolsky, "A large body of evidence suggests that stress-related disease emerges, predominantly, out of the fact that we so often activate a physiological system that has evolved for responding to acute physical emergencies but we turn it on for months on end, worrying about mortgages, relationships, promotions."[3]

What happens to our bodies when we activate the stress response for real or imagined disasters? According to Sapolsky, "Glucose and the simplest forms of proteins and fats come pouring out of your fat cells, liver, and muscles, all to stoke whichever muscles are struggling to save your neck."[4] Our heart rate, breathing, and blood pressure increase, while our sex drive plummets, and digestion is inhibited. Also, immunity to disease is jeopardized.[5]

While our immune system is "enhanced" or temporarily stimulated during *brief* stress—stress that lasts an hour or less—prolonged stress has the opposite effect.[6] In fact, Sapolsky states that prolonged stress suppresses the immune system, that marvelous system with its lymphocytes and monocytes (white blood cells), its macrophages, T helper cells, and circulating natural killer cells (NK cells). While these "good guys" begin to be suppressed during prolonged stress, the bad guys— glucocorticoids and other hormones—are secreted in abundance. Sapolsky writes, "During stress it is logical for the body to shut down long-term building projects in order to divert energy for more immediate needs—this inhibition includes the immune system, which, while fabulous at spotting a tumor that will kill you in six months or making antibodies that will help you in a week, is not vital in the next few moments' emergency."[7]

How do the bad guys shut down the good guys? Sapolsky suggests that these arch villains, the glucocorticoids, can shrink the thymus gland, make lymphocytes less responsive to infection, inhibit the release of key messengers in the immune system—the interleukins and interferons—and even kill lymphocytes.[8] In other words, during periods of prolonged stress, glucocorticoids cause the immune system to cease and desist in the task of providing maximal protection, particularly in tumor surveillance. That's when bad things can happen to good people.

BUT ARE STRESS AND CANCER LINKED?

Even though the effects of stress on illnesses such as colds and flu are well documented in medical literature, I found no direct link between stress and cancer as I pored over the research. But I did discover a pattern: Chronic stress leads to depression, which suppresses the immune system, and a suppressed immune system is linked to cancer. For example, separation and divorce, which trigger chronic stress and depression, suppress the immune system. In fact, women who were tested within a year of their separation or divorce had lower percentages of helper T lymphocytes and NK (natural killer) cells.[9] This is serious, since NK cells—that first line of defense against cancer and its recurrence—are particularly vulnerable to loneliness, stress, and depression. We want to keep those NK cells active and happy! Other groups who have shown immune suppression as a result of chronic stress are caregivers for Alzheimer's patients, married men with poor relationships with their wives and others, and women who are unhappily married.[10]

Dr. Robert Maunder, a psychiatrist at the University of Toronto's Mt. Sinai Hospital, is conducting research on stress and illness. In a conversation with him, I suggested that chronic stress, while not *the* cause of cancer, is certainly one of the major factors involved, and he agreed. Then he added, "Researchers have generally attempted to measure something called major life events when looking for a connection between stress and disease. These can be counted. Chronic stress is simply hard to measure."[11]

Even in the research on the link between major life events, depression, and cancer, the results are inconsistent. Some studies find no connection at all; others do. One study by C. Maddock and C. M. Pariante of Maudsley Hospital in London reviewed medical research between 1996 and 2000 and found evidence supporting a link between stress and the onset of major depression, as well as a poorer prognosis in both cardiovascular disease and cancer.[12] Other studies have discovered that women with breast cancer report they experienced severe and major stressors in the five to eight years preceding their diagnosis. According to Dr. Maunder, "Women with breast cancer *already* believe there's a connection between stress, depression, and cancer."[13]

One study by C. C. Chen and his colleagues examined 119 women, ages twenty to seventy, who were seen at breast-cancer outpatient clinics at King's College Hospital in London and later referred for a biopsy if they had a suspicious breast lesion. Of the 119, 41 had breast cancer. The researchers found a connection between "severe life events" in the preceding five years and breast cancer.[14] Another study by A. J. Ramirez and his colleagues compared 50 breast-cancer patients who had experienced a recurrence with 50 who had not. Those who suffered a relapse had experienced many more major adverse life stresses *postdiagnosis* than those who were successfully keeping the disease at bay.[15] The bottom line? Once you're diagnosed with cancer, it is imperative that you reduce, eliminate, and manage sources of stress, particularly chronic stress. Eliminate? Yes, we can sometimes rearrange our lives and eliminate sources of chronic stress. And when we can't? We can reframe the situation, see the positives, or get help.

ATTACHMENT, STRESS, AND CANCER

Of course, not all of us react to stress the same way. What's stressful to one person is benign to another. So people with similarly stressful situations can have different physical responses: One may get cancer or another disease, while another has excellent health. What causes this crucial difference?

Much of the research I reviewed fails to address the emotional or attachment history of the person who is subsequently diagnosed with cancer. Granted, this would be difficult to test; researchers would have to interview children and then follow them for thirty to forty years to correlate early traumas with the later cancers. Yet an article in the *New York Times* states, "Severe stress in early life appears to cast a long shadow."[16] As a psychologist who has treated patients, I know this is true. Understanding our early lives and our attachments to our parents is crucial to realizing who we are now and how we cope with stress. Clinical psychologist Lydia Temoshok, director of the behavioral medicine program at the University of Maryland, believes that a child learns to cope with traumatic events, stress, and family interactions based on the cues he receives from his parents. "Children are prone to develop behaviors that ensure their survival, which usually means making one's parents happy or at least not angry or likely to abandon the child."[17] Temoshok, who has done extensive research on melanoma patients and people with HIV, suggests that those who later develop cancers learn as children to handle stress by ignoring fatigue or pain. They then do the same thing psychologically, ignoring "loneliness, sadness, fear" to keep from antagonizing their parents or being a "burden" to them.[18]

As a psychologist who specialized in attachment research, I know that children who start life with secure, loving emotional bonds with sensitive parents are simply more resilient in the face of adversity than those who were rejected, abused, abandoned, or neglected. This truth is evident early on: Even preschoolers who are securely attached to their parents are popular with peers and display greater tolerance for frustration than those who are insecure. Those without secure attachments are often loners with little tolerance or resilience when experiencing life's problems and often fall apart when stressed.

Think what this means later in life. Emotional insecurity translates into greater loneliness and less resilience in handling the exigencies of life. Also it relates to feeling out of control in noxious situations. Those of us who fall into this category not only get stressed more easily than others, but we have a stronger physiological reaction to stress. For example, Dr. Charles Nemeroff, a psychiatrist at Emory University, and his colleagues found that women who experienced physical or sexual abuse in childhood "secreted more of two stress hormones in response to a mildly stressful situation than women who had not been abused."[19] Not only do we have a stronger physiological response to stress, but we may also be perversely tolerant of chronic stress, refusing to make the life changes needed to stay healthy. After all, we learned early on that our efforts to get what we needed would be either ignored or rebuffed. For some of us this bred a sense of helplessness and depression. We learned either to live without comfort or to take care of ourselves, becoming compulsively self-reliant.

Loneliness and Cancer

Research has shown that many women who develop breast cancer not only have experienced losses and chronic stress but also feel a deep and pervasive sense of loneliness. One study of 826 women awaiting mammograms at a breast clinic found that those in the newly diagnosed cancer group had significantly more loneliness than those in the cystic and normal breast groups.[20] Those who were the sickest were also the most emotionally repressed. In addition, the newly diagnosed cancer group had experienced more profound life stresses, with significantly more women reporting the death of a spouse or close family member in the preceding two years.

A recent study conducted at George Washington School of Medicine by psychiatrist Karen Weihs and Diane Blyler found that women with early stage breast cancer were more likely to die if they had suffered severe stress during the year before their diagnosis. Researchers tracked eighty patients over a seven-year period, starting within a year of their diagnosis. Among the eighty, there were twenty recurrences and fifteen deaths.

The women, all diagnosed with stage 2 cancer that had *not* metastasized to their lymph nodes, filled out questionnaires about their lives. The women who had severe stress—a family death, a divorce, a financial crisis, a son with HIV—were more likely to die. In fact, severe stress in the year before diagnosis *tripled* a woman's odds of having a recurrence or dying from the cancer.

What's going on here? The researchers suggest that while breast cancer is itself hugely stressful, stress in the year before diagnosis renders the body less able to fight the disease. The immune system is simply "maxed out."[21]

What conclusion can we draw? Chronic stress can kill us. It compromises our immune system so that if we develop cancer, we have no more "magic bullets" in our arsenal to combat our deadly disease.

REDUCING CHRONIC STRESS

So how do we reduce chronic stress in our lives? The key is to feel we have some control over the cause of this stress.

First, we need to identify all those areas of stress that make us feel helpless or hopeless. Take time to thoroughly examine your life. Look beyond the obvious sources of stress—money worries, job problems, time pressures. What else is troubling you or eroding your peace? Is it a difficult, corrosive, enmeshed family relationship? A lack of purpose in life and a sense of drifting aimlessly through the years? Deep-seated loneliness and feeling that you can't connect with anyone? A sense of being trapped as the major or primary family breadwinner? Be honest with yourself, and write down your sources of stress. I suggest you complete this exercise over several days to truly analyze what's happening in your life.

Next ask: How can I change? If you're working at a stressful job you hate, can you quit, go part time, or find another job? If your house payments are too high, can you sell your house and scale down to a simpler home? If your marriage is painful and draining, will your spouse commit to weekly counseling sessions? If your life is joyless, can you add some life-affirming activities, like joining a gardening club, taking horseback-riding lessons, or regularly playing tennis? If you carry your adult children's burdens, failures, or health problems too close to your chest, can you get professional help to create healthier boundaries? After all, they're adults and get to make their own choices just as you did at their age. You are no longer responsible for their successes and failures.

Finally, make an effort to understand yourself and how you cope with stress. Commit to positive life change (see chapter 11, "Emotions and Cancer"). Obviously, we can't eliminate all sources of chronic stress; some stress is nonnegotiable. You can't abandon a sick parent or child, nor would you want to. But you can reframe the situation and imbue it with meaning and purpose. I'm watching a close friend care for her only daughter, a lovely thirty-four-year-old who has had ALS for almost four years. The daughter can hardly move, she's on a feeding tube, and her mother struggles to understand her words. Yet my friend and her daughter possess a deep faith in God, and my friend is committed to making life pleasurable for her child and herself. Both find meaning and purpose in a tragic circumstance. My friend tells me God will give them strength and grace for whatever lies ahead.

You can also enlist family members, caregivers, and friends for ongoing help so that you can rest. Moreover, you can set boundaries and enforce them with an out-of-control child. And you can say no to commitments that sap your strength and consume too much energy.

IS CHANGE POSSIBLE?

Remember Rachael, who felt that rats were nibbling her to death? She quit her job in San Francisco and started her own investment firm, working from home. She is basking in her new freedom and reduced stress. Recently she told me, "I just love to cut the first business deal of the morning in my pajamas."

Julie, who discovered she had breast cancer after her husband's death, also made positive changes. When the job she took after Jim's death proved toxic, she woke up one morning and said to herself, "I don't have to do this. I don't have to work for this impossible boss anymore." She quit that day and discovered in the weeks ahead that another, less stressful job was waiting for her. Today she loves her life and says, "I went through so much in those years when Jim was dying that I learned how strong I am. I can't imagine that I'll ever have to deal with that much stress again."

What happened to Leona when she found out she had melanoma? Not only did she work on her marriage and find a new career, but she turned to her girl-friends for emotional support. "My girlfriends are my lifeline," says this woman who every year travels to Colorado, where she grew up, to spend several days with women who have been her close friends since the ninth grade—for thirty-three years! Her friends, who know the intimate details of her life, are not only tremendous stress reducers but great fun to be with as well.

Leona, who earlier described herself as "a beautiful bird almost dying in a cage," now says she is an eagle. "I am strong. I can fly. I no longer need negative stuff in my life." Now better able to manage life's inevitable stresses, Leona says she tries to live in the moment, to be "vitally alive." She told me, "Girl, I live life at full speed!"

PRACTICAL HELP FOR REDUCING STRESS

If you need some help in getting a handle on stress, let me suggest some simple steps to get you started.

- *Reframe the way you view stress.* Work to change negative perceptions into positive ones. For example, you may choose to view caring for a sick parent as an honor, rather than a daily drudgery. Or you might view mending a difficult relationship as a chance to restore something that's important.
- *Talk to close friends about your stresses.* Their warmth and empathy will enable you to relax and cope, and their suggestions may help you make positive changes.
- *Find a therapist, minister, or priest to talk to regularly.* Sometimes we need a neutral, wise professional to offer insights and solutions. Therapy, for example, is a wonderful venue to say all the things we wouldn't dream of saying to our friends and family. A neutral professional can also recommend new strategies for handling our lives and provide support as we

implement them. Therapy also helps with the enmeshed family relationships that those of us with cancer tend to have.

- *Dedicate an hour each day to relaxation and self-care.* This may be time to take a luxurious bubble bath, read just for pleasure, lie in front of a cozy fire, take a walk, or use your creative gifts. Whatever you do, make sure this time is really for you: answering e-mails, making the next day's lunches, and washing the car don't count.

- *Eat a nutritious diet, and get plenty of rest.* Food and sleep should be non-negotiable; they're important for both your physical health and emotional well-being. Turn food preparation into a fun part of your day by playing your favorite CDs and involving friends and family in creating meals and fresh juices.

- *Plan a vacation to escape from stress.* Do what you enjoy, whether it's sightseeing, walking on the beach, or playing golf. Use vacation time to escape from your problems and rediscover your relaxed self. You'll be better able to make life changes when you return.

- *Take up an enjoyable new hobby* you've always wanted to explore. Practice fly-fishing, take a Pilates class, or join a gardening club. Learn a new skill, like speaking French, cooking Vietnamese food, or painting watercolors.

- *Fill your mind with inspiring stories,* like those in *Guideposts.* As you read the first-person accounts of how people have conquered disease, survived natural disasters, or transformed lost lives with God's help, you will get a sense of God's larger plan. Equally important, you'll build your faith in his ability to work miracles when situations are bleak.

- *Spend time each day reading the Bible and praying.* The psalms are great stress reducers, and prayer slows the heart rate and calms our mind. We can pray alone or with other people and experience less anxiety and greater peace.

- *Go to church more than once a week.* Join a care group, take a course in spiritual gifting or church history, or volunteer to teach a class. Being more involved in the life of your church will help you feel less lonely and stressed and more connected to other people. And as you hear about other people's struggles, you'll feel more optimistic about your own. God created us for community.

- *Play with small children.* Children have a remarkable ability to anchor us in the present and teach us joy in life's small things. And it's so fulfilling to bring happiness to a small child, whether you're playing chase, swinging your small friend, or practicing a jump shot.

RESIGN AS MANAGER OF THE UNIVERSE

At a stimulating conference at the Blue Ridge Assembly in Asheville called Medicines from the Earth, I heard Donald Yance speak about stress and adrenal burnout. He said, "The typical American lifestyle today is one of frantic time schedules, fast food, sedentary work, and chronic high stress. It all seems so mundane, meaningless, and often nonhuman. Many, if not all, chronic health conditions are in some way related to long-term stress."[22]

To live a more balanced life, we have to stop frenetically running and doing. Instead, we must examine our lives and change our priorities. Larry Burkett told me that he finally escaped from the vortex of chronic stress when his son Dan was in an automobile accident and lay in a coma for three months. During the weeks he sat by his son's bedside, Larry examined his life and changed his priorities. "As I focused on my son and his recovery, I realized that other things just weren't as important," said Larry. "One of the smarter things I did was get a tax attorney, give him power of attorney, and turn the IRS guy over to him. I should have done that earlier, but I tend to think I can solve all my problems." Then with some humor, he added, "Basically, I resigned as God's manager of the universe."[23]

Larry died on July 4, 2003, of congestive heart failure—cancer free. He was a true cancer warrior, because, other than Larry, "of the seventy area patients treated for the same cancer at the same time, all were dead within two years."[24] According to a September 2002 letter sent out by Terry Parker, chairman of the board for Crown Financial Ministries, after Larry's diagnosis he asked the Lord for eight more years to "prepare the ministry for his homegoing." He lived an additional eight years and four months.

Larry and Rachael and Julie and Leona chose to change their lives once they discovered they had cancer. What about you? Why not choose to reclaim your lost power and reinvent yourself and your life?

EMOTIONS AND CANCER

Old traumas don't die, but unlike old soldiers, they don't fade away either. Unless you take steps to undo them, they stick with you like wall-paper.

DR. HAROLD BLOOMFIELD

We know that the mind, or the brain, is the master regulator of the body. We can work with our minds to improve conditions in the body so that cancer meets more resistance to developing and growing.

ALASTAIR CUNNINGHAM

I've seen some people, as they've resolved some of the places where they've been [psychologically] stuck in their lives, live better and far longer than anyone would have expected.

DR. JAMES GORDON

In April 1985 Dr. Alice Epstein's physician told her that she had kidney cancer and that it had spread to her lungs. His prognosis? The cancer was incurable. How long did she have to live? "Well, in cases like this, where cancer has spread in the lung and is probably growing in the primary area as well, I'd say about three months," replied the oncologist.[1]

Alice's response? "I gasped for air as I heard him reply, and I kept saying to myself, 'So this is what it is to be. This is what it is to be. Oh no!' "[2] She started sobbing. Although Alice's doctor suggested that she get waitlisted for an experimental interferon program at the Yale–New Haven Clinic, he held out little hope.

While she waited to be accepted into the program, Alice decided to work on personality integration with her husband, a clinical psychologist, and Dorothy

(Didi) Firman, a therapist who specializes in psychosynthesis, a spiritually based approach to personality wholeness. What was Alice's goal, given her bleak situation? As her husband, Dr. Seymour Epstein, explained, "She was not trying so much to defeat the cancer but to become the person she wanted to be, not someone whom she believed others wanted her to be."[3] Alice worked hard and, according to her husband, became more "appreciative, loving, assertive and self-accepting." She also became more open as she overcame her unresolved anger and anxiety. As Alice began to change psychologically, she also changed physically. Alice, who never used to sweat, began to perspire when she exerted herself, indicating better bodily functioning. But the most compelling evidence of physiological change was yet to come.

Before the first interferon treatment, Alice had a chest x-ray at the Yale–New Haven Clinic to provide a baseline evaluation. After only a month of intensive psychotherapy, her tumors had shrunk dramatically. Not surprisingly, she decided to postpone the interferon treatment. Her healing continued; shortly thereafter Alice was cancer free. The chief oncologist said "he had never seen a case like Alice's in the history of the Yale–New Haven Clinic."[4]

Clearly, something remarkable had happened.

Four years after her diagnosis Alice wrote about her story in *Mind, Fantasy and Healing*. After I read her book, on impulse I called Alice in Amherst and discovered that this woman, who had cancer at fifty-seven, is now a vibrant, healthy seventy-two-year-old. When I asked her if she ever worried about a recurrence of cancer—something I thought about almost every day during that time—she replied, "No, I worry about osteoporosis." I laughed out loud. I loved hearing those words. Alice had definitely moved on. There was life after cancer.[5]

Later that day I also telephoned her husband at the University of Massachusetts, where he teaches. He told me, "Alice cannot remember the woman she was before she had cancer. Through intensive psychotherapy she has learned to give and receive love. Basically, she learned to love herself."[6]

THE MIND MATTERS

If Alice's work on personality integration and her subsequent recovery sounds far-fetched to you, you should know that researchers have long since established the connection between cancer and personality. In *Cancer As a Turning Point,* Lawrence LeShan writes that until 1900 it was widely accepted in medical circles that psychological factors were linked to the later development of cancer. Usually those who developed cancer had experienced "great emotional loss and hopelessness" before the first indications of cancer appeared. In 1885 surgeon Willard Parker wrote, "It is a fact that grief is especially associated with the disease."[7] Years earlier Sir James Paget stated in his book *Surgical Pathology:*

> The cases are so frequent in which deep anxiety, deferred hope and disappointment are quickly followed by the growth and increase of cancer, that we can hardly doubt that mental depression is a weighty additive to the other influences favoring the development of the cancerous constitution.[8]

Today there's a booming field of research called psychoneuroimmunology, or PNI, that examines the relationship between stress, personality, emotions, and the immune system. Although PNI was once considered a fringe area, since the seventies, research in the field of psychoneuroimmunology has discovered links between the mind (psycho), the nervous system (neuro), and the cells (immunology) of our bodies.[9]

Candace Pert, author of *Molecules of Emotion* and professor of pharmacology at Georgetown University, discovered in her research that our emotions constantly communicate with cells throughout the body via neuropeptides (the biochemical parallels of emotion). The brain releases these neuropeptides, which then attach to cell receptor sites and produce all kinds of cellular changes. According to Pert, "Your mind is in every cell of your body."[10] She believes that our moods and attitudes, which come from "the realm of the mind, transform themselves into the physical realm through the emotions."[11] In other words, our emotions are "a bridge between the mind and the body."[12]

Pert suggests that a growing body of literature, most of it European, shows that our emotional history greatly influences our health. "For example, it appears that suppression of grief and suppression of anger, in particular, are associated with an increased incidence of breast cancer in women."[13] According to Yugoslavian psychotherapist Ronald Grossarth-Maticek, who administered questionnaires to 1,353 people and followed them for a decade, nine out of every ten cases of cancer can be predicted on the basis of "an overly rational, anti-emotional attitude and a tendency to ignore signs of poor health."[14] In the longest study yet, begun in 1946 at Johns Hopkins University, Pirkko Graves and her colleagues followed 972 medical students for three decades and found that loners who suppressed their painful emotions beneath a "bland exterior" were sixteen times more likely to develop cancer than those who openly expressed their feelings.[15]

In an article on the foundations of mind-body medicine, Pert and her colleagues suggest:

> We banish socially unacceptable and/or exceedingly painful emotions
> from consciousness when we are helpless to change conditions that
> cause ongoing stress, anguish, rejection, abandonment, hunger or physical discomfort.[16]

But we pay a high price, as the cancer research shows, when we suppress our painful feelings. Pert and her colleagues ask: "Is it possible that the symptoms of diseases of a compromised mind-body system—the infections, chronic pains, autoimmune disorders, even the cancers—are, in part, messages to the *chronic repressor* that his or her defense is no longer serving to protect well-being?"[17] (emphasis added).

I believe many illnesses are a red alert, telling us to pay attention to our grief, our anger, our pain, our unmet emotional needs. We continue to suppress these powerful emotions at great peril. If we're locked in depression, we need to get help to overcome feelings of helplessness, hopelessness, and hostility. If we're anxious, we need to find outlets for these intense and scary feelings. If terrible things happened to us in childhood, we must end the silence and finally work through what is locked in our brain and in our cells.

Suppression of our anger and grief is no longer an option if we want to survive cancer. It may have been defensive behavior for us as children if we had abusive or alcoholic or neglectful parents, or it may be learned behavior because our wounded parents owned all the anger and rage in our house, refusing to allow us to honestly express our fear, sadness, and anger. But suppression has helped to make us sick. To get well, we need to learn how to appropriately express, rather than suppress, our emotions.

Excavating Our Emotional History

What has caused those of us with cancer to grow up repressing our painful emotions? The key lies in understanding our emotional histories. Starting in the first year of life—between six and twelve months—each of us forged, or tried to forge, an emotional bond, an attachment relationship, with our parents. This emotional bond was either secure or insecure, based on the way our parents treated us.

If they were warm, loving, and responsive to our physical and emotional needs, then we developed a sense of emotional security—a pervasive and enduring sense that we were loved and lovable. Worthy. Moreover, we learned our first lessons about intimacy from our mothers or primary caregivers. And these lessons about love and closeness permeate all of our later love relationships. Freud wrote in *Outline of Psychoanalysis* that a child's relationship with his mother is unique, without parallel, established unalterably for a lifetime as the first and strongest love object and the prototype for all later love relationships for both sexes.[18]

But what if our parents were unloving, unaffectionate, and unresponsive to our needs? What if they were rejecting, neglectful, depressed, or too often physically or emotionally absent? Then we most likely developed a deep and abiding sense of emotional insecurity. Today we may struggle with self-worth and feel unlovable to the core of our being.

Attachment Gone Awry

One woman who later developed melanoma had a mother who was given to bouts of depression and rage, so much so that the daughter spent all her free time at her girlfriends' homes. A man recovering from bladder cancer said his mother often belittled his dad and was frequently depressed and lonely. She was so troubled, in fact, she attempted suicide when he was seventeen years old. Another man told me he could not recall that his father, an investment banker, ever hugged him or told him he loved him. One woman who had thyroid cancer over a decade ago had a mentally ill mother who allowed her daughter no life outside of the house. And a former client in her thirties who found out she has an aggressive breast cancer told me, "My mother was unable to nurture me. Even now she is unable to provide the emotional support I need as I recover from this disease."

One of the saddest stories I have heard was of a woman diagnosed with ovarian cancer who, after she lost her hair because of chemo, was asked by her doctor about the numerous tiny scars on her head. Had she been in a car accident or undergone cranial surgery? She replied that when she was a child, her mother had used a high heel shoe to discipline her, striking her on the head where no one could see the wounds or scars.

Lack of nurture. Parental suicide. Abuse. Our parents gave us what they had to give, and sometimes what they gave was horrendous. But we cannot get stuck in blame and bitterness. We must understand the source of our crippling self-perceptions, lack of self-love, and difficulty in trusting others so we can be healed emotionally, which will, in turn, affect us physiologically.

And if we weren't emotionally close to at least one loving, affectionate parent, we most likely have a deep and pervasive sense of loneliness, which research has linked to breast cancer (see chapter 10, "Chronic Stress and Cancer"). But loneliness knows no gender barrier, affecting both men and women deeply. And this lack of intimacy with others keeps us from feeling or experiencing the love and support we so desperately need, both before and after cancer.

LARRY BURKETT'S STORY

When I interviewed Larry Burkett, the well-known Christian author and financial counselor, he told me that his metastasized renal cell carcinoma had recurred three times, the last time in his brain. He indicated that he was not afraid and that he had always viewed cancer as a "project." He was at peace with himself, unafraid of death because, as he said, "I know where I'll spend eternity." He added, "I just don't like the process of cancer; it's so expensive and time-consuming."

After we discussed the years of chronic stress leading up to his diagnosis of cancer, I asked him if he had been emotionally close to his parents, both of whom are now deceased. The fifth of eight children, Larry told me that he had "no relationship" with his father, a workaholic. "I played sports all my life, and he never came for a single game. My mother was a chronic hypochondriac, and the Great Depression had a huge impact on her. Although my father was an electrician and made a decent living, she always thought she was poor."

Although he said he loved his mother and got to know her well in her later years, Larry told me, "I never heard her say a kind word about another human being. I stayed away from home as much as was humanly possible when I was growing up. My siblings? We were never close; we were not a family."

An admitted workaholic himself, Larry was determined to become a different kind of father to his children, and he either coached or attended his children's games as they were growing up. But he said that he always struggled with intimacy, both with his wife and children. When he married, he was nineteen, and his wife was only sixteen. "I was driven to succeed," Larry said. "With me, with my personality, closeness is very, very difficult." Larry, who admitted he struggled with loneliness, added that when he got hurt, his tendency was to withdraw. "I found I could withdraw into myself and get along."

Fortunately for Burkett, his relationships had begun to change in recent years. When we spoke, he said that he was emotionally closer than ever to his wife and children. Also, he had experienced the joy of pouring his life into his grandchildren, even helping to raise a grandson, who, along with his divorced mother, lived in Larry's home for eleven years. "My grandson and I are extremely close," said Larry.[19]

Larry's candid commentary corresponds with what the research has found to be true for those of us who struggle with cancer. Namely, that we were not close to our parents in childhood, and we carry these first lessons about love and intimacy into all our later intimate relationships. Yet the healing of childhood wounds is not only possible but necessary if we are to have the best chance of reclaiming our health. We need to be close to others to be able to receive essential emotional and practical support for the journey ahead. According to Dr. James Gordon, "If we have people we're close to—they could be professionals, family members, friends—then epidemiological studies show we're likely to do better once we have cancer and live longer."[20]

Not only does our emotional history affect our capacity for intimacy, but it affects the way we cope with stress as well.

THE TYPE C COPING STYLE

One clinical psychologist who has become internationally known for her groundbreaking research on cancer patients and stress is Dr. Lydia Temoshok. Her research has shown an important link between changing ineffective patterns of coping with stress and increasing one's odds of long-term survival.

In 1979, Dr. Temoshok was asked by the directors of the melanoma clinic at the University of California, San Francisco, to conduct research on their patients. Some were doing better than expected, while others were doing worse than expected. The doctors suspected that psychological and stress factors were responsible, as recovery didn't always correlate to the severity of the melanoma. "Some people with thin lesions did badly," said Dr. Temoshok, "while others with thick lesions did well."

Dr. Temoshok began interviewing the melanoma patients to discover how they were coping with their illness. "What was immediately striking was that nearly everyone we interviewed was much different from individuals who have the Type A coping style that typifies the people prone to heart disease. Those folks are quick to anger; they're very impatient and focused on themselves," she said. "The melanoma patients, on the other hand, were focused on other people, and they didn't seem to remember a time in their lives when they were ever angry." Temoshok called the behavior of these cancer patients the Type C coping style.

According to Temoshok, the Type C coping style refers to the way the individual copes with stress. "The most critical factor, the one most often linked to problems with the immune system, is that the person is not focused on himself. He doesn't seem to pay attention to signals from his own body—his emotional cues—particularly anger or sadness." She added, "Emotions are there to protect us; they're adaptive. We get angry if somebody is abusing us. We get sad because there's a situation where we're losing something." Type Cs tend to say that "everything is okay" and ignore emotional signals to the contrary. Their chief worry? What other people think. "They focus on what does everyone else want them to be: together, strong, pleasant, nice," said Temoshok.

This lack of self-awareness and failure to pay attention to emotional cues is particularly salient in stressful situations. According to Temoshok, Type Cs don't always realize they're under stress, so they stay in stressful situations far too long. "If they have a boss who says, 'I want you to stay late every night this week,' they don't say, 'Am I getting paid extra for this?' Nor do they recognize their feelings of anger. They just stay late and do the work. Because of this, they make great employees," she added. But this tendency to stay in stressful situations too long without attending to or expressing their emotions gets Type Cs in trouble physiologically and leads to the suppression of their immune systems.

How the Type C Coping Style Develops

I asked Dr. Temoshok how cancer patients develop the Type C coping style in the first place. "It starts when you're a kid. Now this is all theoretical; we don't have any data on this. But there's plenty of data from other sources on how children or young animals learn coping patterns that are not just psychological but are biological as well," Temoshok said. "If you have parents who don't support the expression of emotions and say, 'Big boys don't cry' or 'I don't want to ever hear you express anger' or 'I don't have time for this,' you learn not to bother your parents but rather to suppress your feelings. Then you learn to pay attention to the parent because the parent determines how you 'should' feel."

Temoshok told me that a large number of "the severe Type Cs" she has worked with have been abused, either physically, sexually, or emotionally. Because they grew up in perilous situations, these future Type Cs developed a coping style that enabled them to survive. "But this coping style doesn't serve them well in adulthood," said Temoshok. Consequently, she tries to help them understand they can finally talk about their painful emotions, the jobs they hate, their difficult marriages. "Because Type Cs are so interested in pleasing everyone, they don't stop to ask themselves if they're happy or not," she explained.

So how can Type Cs change their coping style to increase their chance of survival? According to Dr. Temoshok, first of all, the cancer patient must learn to recognize signs of stress in his own body. This is no easy task since Type Cs have been shut down to emotional cues in childhood. To help her clients develop self-awareness, Dr. Temoshok says, "I do whatever it takes." She described hooking up patients to blood pressure machines, skin conductor machines, even lie detectors to show them how their emotions are affecting them physiologically. She tells her cancer patients, "Look, this is what happens when you're asked to do something you know in your heart you don't want to do, and yet you're saying out loud, 'Oh yes, I'll do that.' Look what's happening to your blood pressure." The patient is usually calm at that point, so the psychologist presses further. "What's going to happen to your body if you do this ten to twenty times a day?"

Temoshok's goal? She tries to teach cancer patients to become more attuned to their emotional responses and to stop repressing and ignoring their feelings. Temoshok believes that cancer patients need to change their difficult situations or get out of them. "Sometimes they need to quit that job or end that destructive relationship, and people who are able to do this have experienced remarkable changes in their health." She added, "Our research has shown that the more you change your maladaptive Type C coping behavior, the better your prognosis will be."

In addition to recognizing Type C behavior, Temoshok helps cancer patients acquire new interpersonal skills to resolve stressful situations. Most need to become more assertive, but sometimes when they say no, they become so aggressive that it causes problems with their spouse or boss. Because standing up for their own needs is so unfamiliar, they don't understand how to do so appropriately. Since this is often the case, Temoshok teaches her cancer patients scripts for saying no to people. She helps them get their needs met more diplomatically so they will be more effective.

When I asked Dr. Temoshok if people could change their Type C coping behavior without psychotherapy, she responded, "I think it's really, really hard to do that because you're changing a lifelong habit. It's hard to do this even with psychotherapy. I've had some patients say, 'I've done this for fifty years. I have a family, a job, a life, and I can't change.'" Then Dr. Temoshok tells them that while she respects their choices, their decisions may affect their health. Patients usually respond, "I'm sure the research is valid, but I'm choosing to stay the same." When this happens, says Temoshok, the cancer outcome is usually worse than would have been predicted. Sometimes patients die.

Temoshok admits that having patients refuse to change their coping styles has been one of the most discouraging aspects of her work. "What's behind this resistance?" I asked. "Is it all about self-love or self-worth?" Temoshok responded that cancer patients who have been abused have particularly negative self-images. "They don't feel good about themselves," she said. "But I've seen people change their lifelong patterns of thinking and coping with stress, so it can be done."

At the end of our interview, I asked Dr. Temoshok how her research has been received. While she admits that some therapists worry about cancer patients' blaming themselves for getting cancer, Temoshok says she tries to be crystal clear that patients are not to blame for their disease. But the Type C pattern, if used too often over the years in situations where it isn't appropriate, produces excessive secretion of stress hormones and "a consequent down regulation of the immune system. Over time, this makes these individuals not only more vulnerable to getting cancer but also to having it develop more quickly."

Regarding the response of cancer patients themselves, Temoshok said that her research elicits an "aha" from them. "Most say, 'You've described my situation. What can I do to help myself?' or 'You've just described my sister. What can I do to help her?'" She believes that the most positive aspect of her research is that it gives patients the knowledge they need to make powerful, life-affirming changes in their coping styles and their relationships. When cancer patients do make significant changes, they're not only happier and feel better about themselves, but many live longer.[21]

MARABEL'S STORY

One woman who dramatically changed her coping style, self-perceptions, and life is Marabel Morgan. I met Marabel at a National Prayer Breakfast about seven years ago. Eager to see what this lady who wrote *Total Woman* and gave the feminists heartburn was really like, I walked up after the breakfast and introduced myself. Marabel was warm, friendly, and prettier than any woman in her late fifties had a right to be. After our initial conversation, we met again for tea and discovered we had a genuine bond—our mothers. Marabel's relationship with her mother was as painful and encompassing as mine had been, and we both felt we had finally met someone who understood the legacy of mother love gone awry. During the conversation she told me she had had thyroid cancer years earlier; consequently, Marabel was one of the first people I called when I was diagnosed with breast cancer.

Marabel learned she had thyroid cancer fifteen years ago. After surgery to remove the tumor that had spread to her lymph nodes, with fear and trembling she decided to have radiation. She was put in a room by herself and had to take pills contained in a miniature silo, brought in by a hospital employee covered from head to toe. His hand shaking like a leaf, he said, "Here, take these. I'm getting out of here."

During her stay at the hospital, Marabel received food through a tiny opening in the door three times a day. Her room was bare, except for a bed, table, and lamp.

Her connections with the outside world? A window and a telephone. In a corner of her room she found a piece of paper, headed by a picture of a skull and crossbones, that read, "If the patient dies, get a hook and pull him out. Do not, under any circumstances, touch the patient."

Marabel said to herself, "I'm doomed. If cancer doesn't get me, the radiation will." Afraid and depressed, she didn't believe at first that she could beat cancer. In fact, she said, "I gave up. After I got out of the hospital, I saw this sweater I liked, but I didn't buy it. I told myself, you're going to die before you ever wear it out." During the first months after her surgery and radiation, she awoke every morning surprised she was still alive. Her "blue funk" lingered.

When I asked her what was happening in her life prior to cancer, this author, who had been on the cover of *Time* in 1977, said that when her "fifteen minutes of fame" were over, she felt a letdown. "It was like holding on to a tornado. Whatever I did was media worthy. I enjoyed it; it was a hoot," she said, laughing. At the height of the Total Woman wave, Marabel had seventy-two teachers teaching Total Woman seminars in the United States, Germany, and South Africa, and she flew to Japan to speak to eight thousand people. "I didn't take it too seriously, but it was a loss when the phone stopped ringing continually." By 1985 the Total Woman phenomenon was on the wane. Two years later Marabel was diagnosed with cancer.

Marabel admitted she had struggled with depression for as long as she could remember. "Although I was bright and cheerful with Charlie and the girls, I always felt that depression was crouching behind the back door. And when cancer hit, I felt alone in it. The girls were away at school, and I would say to Charlie, 'Take me in your arms and hold me.' I was trembling inside. Although Charlie was responsive, he couldn't hold me on the inside where I was constantly shaking. I finally realized that Jesus was the only one who could hold me inside. That helped enormously."

Marabel's struggle with depression had its roots in her relationship with her mother, who cut off all ties with her daughter when she became a Christian at age twenty-three. "All of my adult life," says Marabel, "I was looking for her, hoping to be reunited. I would go to her house in Ohio, ring the bell, and call out, 'Mom.' She never opened the door. I felt crushed, abandoned, rejected." Marabel's mother, who died recently, never met Marabel's husband or her two daughters, both of whom are married and have children themselves. She did not see Marabel for almost forty years. Once Marabel's younger daughter, Michelle, drove to Ohio while she was in college, knocked on her grandmother's door, and heard a voice inside ask, "Who is it?" "I am your daughter's daughter," Michelle replied. "Go away," her grandmother responded.

For Marabel, her mother's absolute rejection felt like chronic stress, always "there under the surface." Several years after her cancer diagnosis, she went to a counselor who told her, "You've been depressed all of your life." Because Marabel was adept at suppressing her painful emotions, having done it since childhood, she said, "No one knew I was depressed. I didn't even know at a certain level."

Once she began receiving counseling, Marabel recounted her painful childhood, including her father's leaving when she was a baby. Describing her mother, Marabel said, "She was a Dr. Jekyll and Mr. Hyde," who could be "soft and sweet" and turn venomous on a dime. Fortunately, when Marabel was in third grade, her mother married a kind man who loved Marabel. But for some unknown reason, her mother took to her bed for six years and controlled the two of them from a room she never left.

Marabel's stepfather died when she was in the ninth grade. "Mother kept the blinds drawn all the time, and it was like living in a dark cave," said Marabel of her childhood home, where all the rooms were painted dark green. The darkness penetrated Marabel's mind and heart. With no loving parent at home, school became her only escape. As a ninth grader Marabel would sing on her way to school "Whistle While You Work" or "Pretend You're Happy When You're Blue." By the time she was a senior, she would recite, "I can do everything through him who gives me strength," just to have the courage to go into the school building. Her mother wouldn't allow her to date or accept the college scholarship she rightfully earned.

At age sixteen Marabel went to the downtown courthouse and asked to see a judge. For years her mother had threatened to send the police after her if she ever ran away. So Marabel told the judge, "I want to run away when I'm eighteen. Can my mother force me to return home?" The kindly man looked sadly at her and said, "No, no. When you're eighteen, run, honey, run."

When Marabel did leave her mother's home, she carried with her all those painful memories of maternal rejection and abandonment. It wasn't until she went into counseling after cancer that she began to get free. "Don't you get it?" her counselor asked, leaning toward her. "Your mother doesn't *want* to have a relationship with you." Shocked, Marabel realized he was right and began to release her yearning for a viable relationship with her emotionally crippled mother. This proved to be a turning point in her life and key to her ability to survive cancer.

Today Marabel says that her will to live is strong, and depression no longer crouches at the back door of her mind. Refusing to be trapped in a cycle of rejection, depression, and painful yearning, Marabel today has her own business and is emotionally close to Charlie, her two daughters, and grandchildren. Moreover, she believes God has a plan for her life. "More than anything in the world, I want to live in his will, please him, serve him. This is the main desire of my life. I've been given my assignment: to be a light in the darkness."

The girl who was trapped in a dark house with a mentally ill mother says her life has never been happier. The same woman who once woke up surprised she was still alive says that she now welcomes each new day, stretches, and feels "young and frisky." Not bad for sixty-five and counting.[22]

Finding Peace, at Last

After I read Alice Epstein's book, I felt certain that her therapist, Didi Firman, could help me. For years I had been conscious of how my relationship with an emotionally unstable mother had affected all my intimate relationships and the way I handled stress. Mother had no idea how to love and nurture my sister and me. Moreover, she battled depression and was often hostile and sometimes cruel. That meant I had to stuff my emotional needs as a child and learn how to handle them on my own because I got no help from her. My wounded, narcissistic mother was too wrapped up in her troubles to notice mine.

For years I had yearned to be free from my wounded past, to make peace with my mother. When I finally, at age fifty-nine, sat down on the sofa in Didi's office to confront my inner demons, I felt I was in the presence of a competent, authoritative therapist who could help me do deep, inner work. Didi quickly took charge. "Tell me about yourself," she said as she sat in a chair in front of me, her graying hair pulled back into a neat ponytail. I told her I had been in therapy the year before and had done some good work on difficult relationships but had never really resolved my relationship with my rejecting and abusive mother at an experiential level. Smiling, I said, "I have saved the best for the last."

I told her that I found myself in the difficult position of having to care for my infirm mother even though I felt the toxic mother of childhood existed in every cell of my body. "This is serious," said Didi, who has worked with many cancer patients since the publication of Epstein's book. "You have two mothers. The toxic mother of childhood and the sick woman in the nursing home. Let's work on the former because you have to continue to care for the latter. Close your eyes, and I want you to envision a photograph of you and your mother."

As I closed my eyes I saw in my mind's eye a photograph taken the day I was a mascot at my Uncle Jack's high school graduation. I was about six at the time. Standing in front of a hedgerow at my grandparents' dairy farm, my raven-haired, attractive mother was ramrod straight as she looked at the camera, smiling. I stood in front of her, scowling. Both of us were dressed in gray and white. Mother had donned a slim, gray dress with a white cowl collar that day while I wore a gray robe with a starched, white collar. "Because of your mother's emotional problems, you have never been able to relate to her personality," said Didi. "But you're a Christian. Imagine that her soul could talk to yours. What would she say?"

I imagined my mother asking for forgiveness for all the cruel and hateful things she had ever said and done. As she asked me to forgive her, my lovely mother reached out and hugged me, something she had great difficulty doing. I cried, staying for a moment in that sunny place, feeling that something deep and profound was happening.

At the end of the session, I felt like Jell-O. Before I left that day, Didi suggested that whenever I took a shower, I tell myself that I was washing the toxic mother of childhood out of every cell of my body. "I have found that those who have cancer need some kind of ritual for ridding their bodies of toxic emotions," she said.

As I left her office the next day after a second session, I felt at peace with Mother for the first time in my life. Relaxed, I ran to meet my husband who was strolling down the street toward Didi's office.

I knew my work with Didi had accomplished something wonderful when my mother came to our home for what would be her last visit, weeks before she died. For the first time in my life, I dealt with her in the present and was no longer engaged in an inner dialogue, like the character Gollum in Tolkien's trilogy, *The Lord of the Rings,* a prisoner of the past. The toxic mother of childhood was no more. Through my work with Didi, I had been able to release long-suppressed grief and yearning. For the first time in my life I felt anchored in the present and could focus on the frail mother in my home who, I realized, was slowly and quietly dying.

Mother died a week shy of her seventy-ninth birthday. I was with her in the hospital, working with the doctors and nurses, loving her, attending to her needs. She had had a stroke and was able to say only yes and no in response to questions. Fortunately, she was not in great pain, and on the last day of her life as her kidneys began to fail, she miraculously got back her full range of language. She held court with Don, me, and her favorite nurses. But she quickly tired, and as she began to drift off to sleep, she told me it was better if I left. "Is there anything we need to talk about, Mother?" I asked.

"No, we've said it all," she replied and closed her eyes. At a quarter till nine that evening, her soul took flight.

On the day of Mother's funeral, my sister and I, along with our husbands, spoke to all who came to honor her life. We talked about who she was and the legacy she had bequeathed her children and grandchildren. We were loving but also painfully honest. I spoke about the pain in Mother's life—her personal tragedies, the pain she had inflicted on her family, and the fact that because she was a Christian, she had finally found peace. At last.

That night as I sorted out some of her belongings, I came across a poem Mother had saved, titled "I'm Free." The anonymous author had written:

> Don't grieve for me for I am free
> I'm following the path God laid for me
> If my parting has left a void
> Then fill it up with remembered joy
> Lift up your heart and share with me—
> God wanted me now; he set me free—

It was as if Mother were speaking to me as she winged her way toward heaven—acknowledging that she was free at last. And so was I.

What About You?

What about you? What psychological baggage are you carrying around locked in some dark corner of your heart and mind? What emotional pain have you repressed or barricaded out of sight? As Dr. Gonzalez said during our first telephone conversation, "People can eat all the organic food in the world and take lots of supplements, but if they don't begin to deal with the abuse in childhood, the trauma, the alcoholic parent, or the unhappy marriage, they won't get well. We work with them on nutrition first so that they can get strong enough to deal with the emotional pain in their lives."[23]

Now is the time for soul searching, heart mending, and housecleaning to rid yourself of toxic memories and emotions at a cellular level. For it is in retracing our emotional history, working through the pain, and experiencing the healing of our emotions that we will attain peace of mind. And a mind at peace is able to devote itself fully to the most important work—helping the body get well.

Why We Need Our Friends—and Others

In addition to helping us grow and giving us pleasure and providing aid and comfort, our intimate friendships shelter us from loneliness.

Judith Viorst

We all tend to feel alone in our suffering. I felt a need to share my feelings with those going through a similar experience and to hear theirs.

Margie Levine

Recently I spent a day with my best friend from high school, a woman I had not seen for forty-two years. While our husbands drove off to attend a football game, Nancy and I spent six hours in Biltmore Village, just walking, talking, and shopping, aware that we were engaging in women's talk and female activities—pursuits that would have driven our husbands quietly crazy. This attractive woman with her salt-and-pepper hair and soft brown eyes was as intelligent, warm, and comforting as I remembered her.

As we sat sipping our tea at Chelsea's, I asked her how she remembered us. "We were best friends," said this former college administrator. *Best friends.* I was delighted by Nancy's response since that was the way I also remembered our friendship, and I realized how easy it was to slip back into the pattern of friendship with this woman.

As we talked about our lives, I found myself being uncharacteristically open with Nancy, telling her about my experience with cancer, my current challenges, my inner life. She, whose mother had struggled with uterine cancer, listened with empathy. In the coziness of the tearoom that cold, rainy Saturday afternoon, I remembered a quote from Elsa Walsh, a *Washington Post* reporter, that I had clipped years ago: "Few comforts are more alluring for a woman than the rich, intimate territory of women's talk.… A woman friend will say, 'You are not alone. I have felt that way, too. This is what happened to me.' Home, in other words." How true these words. When we feel we have been heard and accepted in friendship with another woman, we are *home*.

But what about men? Though they need friendships as much as women do, in *Worlds of Friendship*, sociologist Robert Bell wrote that women have more friends than men their whole lives, and their friendships are more open and go deeper.[1] We disclose more than men do when we get together. We run to each other when we are stressed or lonely or need to talk and unburden ourselves with empathic, caring friends. Men, on the other hand, are more likely to talk to the women in their lives or turn on the television while they try to work out their problems. Research shows that while men need their buddies and love to engage in activities with them—like golfing, fishing, or watching spectator sports—they seldom share their intimate struggles with friends.

As I conduct "In the Company of Women" seminars, invariably wives tell me that their husbands seldom share with other men about marital or work problems or struggles with sex or intimacy. When my husband has lunch with a good friend, I ask this man who can talk deeply, "What did you two talk about?" "Oh," says Don reflecting, "the Hebrew course Russ is taking or airplanes or golf." Then I ask, "Did you talk about your wives?" "Not really," he responds. Most married women I know *always* talk to each other about their husbands. See my point?

In my work as a therapist I found, as did my colleagues, that most who came for counseling were women. Talking about problems is simply more natural for females than males. Now this does not mean that men don't need to talk about their worries and concerns, especially when struggling with something as severe as cancer, but it may not feel natural, especially at first. Yet emotional support is just as important for men as women.

What's So Special About Friends?

In *Surviving Cancer*, Margie Levine writes about the rich practical support she received from her friends during and after her treatment. "Friends shopped for groceries, went to the drugstore, drove me to the hospital and to doctor visits, picked up books and tapes from the library, dropped off clothes at the cleaners. After chemo, my husband asked a friend to roast a turkey; it was in the oven when we came home."[2] Early on, she even had friends answer the phone to deal with the myriad well-wishers who called wanting to know how she was doing.

But practical help is only one thing we need in the early days and months of recovery. We also desperately need our friends to listen as we talk about our fears, pain, confusion, feelings of loss, and confrontation with mortality. But this doesn't happen automatically, as I discovered in the early days after my diagnosis.

Although I considered myself rich in friends at the time, I began to see they couldn't possibly understand what I was feeling—the physical weakness, the terror, the confusion, the pain—nor what I was up against in making life-or-death treatment decisions. They lived in the land of the healthy; I had crossed an invisible boundary line into the territory of the sick. Beyond that, because most women are terrified of breast cancer, my diagnosis made me something of a pariah to a few of my postmenopausal friends on hormone replacement therapy. One close friend, who had been on HRT for years, withdrew for a while because my illness ignited her deepest fear. Like her, I had been on HRT. Suppose she, too, got breast cancer? Sensing her withdrawal, I called her and said that I didn't need *more* from her than before, but I certainly didn't need *less*. She listened, confessed her fear, and as a result, we're still emotionally close today.

I was fortunate. For the most part, my friends drew a comforting circle around me. Solicitous, they sent flowers, called to see how I was doing, and several sat through my surgeries with my family, praying for the surgeon and for my speedy recovery. And when I was reeling from the mastectomy, one who had experienced a double mastectomy drove many miles to assure me that Don could handle my changed body, just as her husband had been able to love hers. And she was right.

Among my closest friends, however, one understood better than the rest what I was facing. Eleanor had watched her brave and intelligent mother battle cancer four times, beating the disease until she developed a brain tumor at age eighty-six. Eleanor helped me enormously by "normalizing" the experience—if that's possible— and by telling me how her mother dealt with cancer while at the same time embracing life. Since I had known and admired Ilde, I was grateful her daughter was my friend.

For women, this support of our friends is no trivial contribution. In speaking about the importance of friendship at a Duke University conference on women's health, Dr. Alice Domar said that women with fewer than five close friends were just as likely to die prematurely as those who smoked and had high cholesterol. Then she added, "Women who have breast cancer and fewer than five close friends are 20 percent more likely to die from the disease."[3] Wow! This certainly underscores the importance of our female friendships not only in terms of physical and emotional well-being but longevity as well. And it should be an impetus for many of us to broaden and deepen our ties.

The same holds true for men. They need to reach out to their male friends and enjoy their support and companionship, especially now. My friend Chip was so grateful that one of his medical partners accompanied him and Becky to M.D. Anderson Hospital in Texas when Chip had his surgery. This same friend encouraged Chip to meet him weekly to work out as he was recovering from surgery. Chip later wrote about this important friendship in a national magazine.

BUT WHAT ABOUT OUR SPOUSES?

In addition to our friends, many of us have spouses who provide love, practical support, and comfort when we need it. One seventy-eight-year-old woman wrote this about her experience with breast cancer at age fifty-seven: "My husband of fifty-six years has always been loving and caring and just happy to have me here and well. He still thinks I'm beautiful."[4]

Another breast-cancer survivor, who found her lump when she was thirty-eight, said of her husband, "From day one, my husband, Bruce, has been my strength. He accepted my mastectomy, my hair loss, without blinking an eye. In the hospital he changed my dressings, fixed my drains, fed me. He was known as the man who never left his wife's side. We've been through hell. Together."[5] Several men I interviewed were open about the love and emotional support they received from their wives as they battled cancer.

But no matter how loving our spouses are, they have their own fears and worries, and sometimes they can't share these with us. In addition, their work load increases substantially as they take care of us, the children, the grocery shopping, and the housework. We may be able to help each other, but if we're overwhelmed emotionally or if we never did intimacy well in the first place, we may not. If you're not able to obtain the emotional support you need from your spouse, don't despair. Understand that you're both trying to cope right now, and seek out family, friends, and other cancer survivors who can serve as sounding boards, comforters, and mentors.

When I had pneumonia weeks before I found the lump, my husband became a tender nurse, bringing soup and flowers to my bed, cleaning the house, running errands, calming my fears. This continued, although to a lesser extent, following my surgery. Only months later did Don tell me that he was overwhelmed with fears about the future and that, not wishing to burden me, he had felt very alone in his struggles. But he rose manfully to the occasion. Since then, his care for sick family members has earned him the title "Nurse Betty II," although he bears no resemblance to Renée Zellweger, the original Nurse Betty. He has even taken his act on the road, traveling to Washington, D.C., when Holly was struck with adult chicken pox, and to Chapel Hill when Kristen and her family came down with a virulent flu. Kristen's friends call him "Saint Don" and add that their fathers would not be comfortable in the Nurse Betty II role, but Don merely smiles at their accolades.

WHEN FRIENDS AND SPOUSES ARE NOT ENOUGH

While friends and spouses can give us emotional and practical support in the early days and weeks of our recovery, we also need the company of others who have experienced cancer and are years beyond the diagnosis. These cancer warriors give us hope. They can say with authenticity, "I know how you feel; I've been there too." These men and women are able to relate to us in a way that no spouse, child, or friend can, simply because they, too, have experienced cancer. Once word got out that I had breast cancer, social acquaintances and even strangers called to offer much-needed encouragement and support. One by one, these cancer survivors called to share their stories, their cancer-fighting programs, their faith journeys.

The Importance of Support Groups

While I found support in one person at a time, others, like my friend Shirley, chose to join a support group. Much research has been done on the importance of support groups as a way for cancer patients to combat loneliness, ease suffering, and connect emotionally on the issues that a life-threatening illness raises. One analysis of a number of support-group studies found that participants enjoyed the group process, learned a lot about cancer and its treatment, and experienced less pain as well as improved self-esteem.[6]

Both Dr. Dean Ornish and Dr. Keith Block have included support groups as an integral part of their work with patients. With his heart patients and his prostate cancer patients, Ornish told me that support groups were central in the healing process. Dr. Block also considers support groups an important part of psychosocial support for cancer patients.

One of the most famous studies of the effects of support groups was led by Dr. David Spiegel of the Stanford University School of Medicine, who was initially skeptical about the power of psychological intervention with cancer patients. To test the relevance of support groups, he and his colleagues assigned eighty-six women with metastatic breast cancer to one of two groups: a control group that received only routine oncological care and an experimental group that met weekly for ninety-minute sessions for up to a year. In the experimental group, women learned relaxation techniques and assertiveness and coping skills. They were able to express their feelings honestly and receive support from the group leaders and other women. They were also encouraged to take charge of their lives, to become actively involved in all aspects of their health, to confront their fear of dying. The result? When Spiegel did a follow-up on the two groups after ten years, those in the experimental group had lived twice as long as those in the control group (an average of 36.6 months versus 18.9 months).[7] Moreover, three of the women in the experimental group were still alive after all those in the control group had died.

Another exciting study of melanoma patients (both men and women) by Dr. F. I. Fawzy and his colleagues showed similar results. Dr. Fawzy conducted a study of stage 1 and stage 2 melanoma patients using structured group therapy. The experimental group met in psychotherapy groups of seven to ten patients for ninety minutes weekly for six weeks. During the intervention sessions, the experimental group learned about melanoma, basic nutrition, stress management, and better problem solving and coping skills. In addition, the participants received emotional support from staff and other group members. The control group did not have any psychiatric intervention and did not meet with group leaders.

The original study found that those who participated in the experimental group had higher energy, were more proactive in coping with their illness, and exhibited less depression and higher self-esteem than the control group. Not only did they get crucial ongoing support, but they also got tools to fight their illness. Five years later, when Fawzy and his colleagues did a follow-up study of the original participants, they found that the people in the experimental group were more likely to have survived than those in the control group. Whereas only three of the thirty-four people in the experimental group had died, ten of the thirty-four in the control group had died. Moreover, those individuals who had been openly and honestly distressed at the time of their diagnosis were also more likely to be alive. The researchers suggested that repression of emotion and minimization of the disease had adverse effects, perhaps causing some with cancer to deny the seriousness of their disease and thus fail to make important life-enhancing changes.[8]

The Pathways Program

In exploring the efficacy of support groups, I decided to look at what's happening closer to home. I discovered Dr. Shirley Taffel, a psychologist in her late forties who runs Pathways, a life-after-cancer program, to help men and women with cancer make the radical changes they need to defeat cancer. (While some men participate in the Pathways program, Taffel admits that more women than men come.) She describes her program as "deeper" than a typical support group because she works with clients to "excavate" destructive core beliefs that could sabotage their efforts to get well. As the participants begin to heal their lives and let go of destructive beliefs, their bodies start to recover. In fact, Dr. Taffel told me that of the hundreds of cancer patients she has worked with over the years only two have died.

What's unique about the Pathways program? Dr. Taffel said, "We endeavor to strengthen the immune system because we know that anxiety and depression suppress the immune system. Our aim is to help treatment be as successful as possible to prevent recurrence. To that end, we offer education, psychotherapy, and support."

Dr. Taffel feels that "many of the people who participate in our groups are not comfortable with anger; they've learned to repress their feelings. Basically, they're more caring of others than of themselves. Since one of the characteristics of survivors is assertiveness (and assertiveness is more than being able to take your shoes back if they don't fit), we work on helping our clients become assertive. Assertiveness is all about understanding that you're worthy, you deserve respect, and you are entitled to voice your needs." She added, "Now you may not *get* what you want, but you're entitled to *ask* for what you want."

Dr. Taffel stated that while some who have cancer don't struggle with self-worth, most of the women she works with do. "I see many, many women who have been brought up to believe they should always care for others. In fact, their worth is measured by how much and how well they take care of others." Because of this, Taffel and her staff help patients learn to value themselves as much as they value others—a familiar theme I heard from the physicians and therapists I interviewed and one I tackle in chapter 7, "Nurturing Ourselves." She said that one of the men in the group felt he had to work all the time. He hadn't taken a vacation in seven years. With group support, this individual started to change, to ask for time off so he could begin to enjoy his life.

Dr. Taffel told me she expects her clients to change—their perceptions, their core beliefs, their lives. "People need to examine their lives, their values, and discover what's toxic in their lives. We confront people about their behavior patterns and attitudes because we want them to see cancer as a wake-up call, an opportunity to honestly examine their lives. They've had a brush with death." She paused and said, "You know, most of us believe we're never going to die. As Woody Allen says, 'Most people think death is optional.'"

Changing the Soup

To heal the body, Taffel feels that those with cancer must heal their lives. Influenced by Alastair Cunningham, an internationally known researcher in psycho-oncology and a cancer survivor himself, Taffel has adopted Cunningham's model in her work. According to Cunningham, cancer grows in whatever chemical "soup" the body provides. If someone is an angry person, then, Cunningham believes, cancer has grown accustomed to growing in angry soup. If someone is depressed, then "any cancer that grows to visible size likes depressed soup."[9] To resist cancer, Dr. Cunningham suggests the cancer patient change his "internal soup"—reduce stress, move toward peace of mind, reduce conflict in relationships—so the body ceases to be a cancer host. He adds, "As the mind changes in this way, so it will signal the body that all is well, and the soup will return to a composition that is the best possible for restraining cancer growth—or any other disease for that matter."[10]

To this end, Dr. Taffel and her staff teach clients how to change their "soup" through good nutrition, stress reduction, relaxation techniques, exercise, meditation and prayer, deep breathing, and the honest expression of emotions. Dr. Taffel admits that most cancer patients have a tough time expressing their emotions honestly. "If someone is angry, he or she is encouraged to process this emotion. If someone is sad, we say, 'Go ahead and cry; we'll hold you.' Then the feelings can flow and not get stuck in the body. Basically, we teach people not to stay in a state of turmoil, because of the negative impact on the immune system," she said. Taffel has little patience for the Pollyanna attitude some cancer patients exhibit. She told me, "Unfortunately, they wrongly believe that showing positive feelings while sitting on a powder keg of negative emotions will cure their illness."

Why this recurrent theme of emotional repression? Dr. Taffel believes, at base, that most cancer patients feel unloved and unworthy. That's why they engage in self-destructive behavior, drive themselves relentlessly, and sabotage their health through workaholism and poor nutrition. "At Pathways, we give people permission to love and nurture themselves. We often ask, 'What did you do this week to nurture yourself?' After a period of time, clients begin to say, 'I'm finally learning to love myself.' For many with cancer, this is a strange and wonderful admission."

At the end of our conversation, Dr. Taffel told me about a client—we'll call her Karen—who had come to Pathways the year before with an aggressive form of colon cancer that had metastasized to her liver, prompting her oncologist to give her a bleak prognosis. Taffel began working on the woman's core beliefs in earnest. Karen's mother had lost her parents in a plane crash months before Karen was born. "Her mother was devastated and afraid she would also lose her children. She was so anxious that my client grew up obsessing about her health because she had an unconscious belief she would die young," said Taffel. Then Karen's sister died when Karen was ten years old, so she came to believe she didn't deserve to live. "These were unconscious beliefs excavated during the group process," said Taffel. "The patient didn't realize she had been given a death message by her mother, who was depressed when my patient was born. She had learned to carry her mother's grief and sorrow in her own body. But because she had the courage to share her story with us, she was finally able to work through her grief and realize she didn't need to die just because her sister had." As I stood to go, Taffel said, "Today this woman is in remission and her oncologist is amazed."[11]

Family, friends, cancer warriors, support groups—we may need them all as we struggle to reclaim our health. Centuries ago the British poet John Donne wrote, "No man is an island." Each of us who struggles with cancer knows just how true these words are.

DEALING WITH
DIFFICULT PEOPLE

*If you can't tell the truth in your relationships, they're not relationships—
they're arrangements.*

CHERYL RICHARDSON, life coach

*Without forgiveness life is governed by an endless cycle of resentment and
retaliation.*

ROBERTO ASSAGIOLI

It was nine o'clock at night as I sat in bed reading and half listening to my
favorite, soothing CD when the phone rang. "Hello," I said sleepily.

A female voice responded, "Hi, my name is Tracy, and I'm calling from Indi-
ana. I got your phone number from a mutual friend, who said you might be able
to help me. I was diagnosed with breast cancer, and whatever treatment options I
choose, I also want to go the nutritional route. Do you have a few minutes to talk
to me now?"

"Sure," I said, putting my book aside and sitting up a little straighter. "Tell me
about your situation."

The woman then told me she was in her second marriage and that she and her
husband had custody of his daughter. According to Tracy, the seventeen-year-old
was rebellious, insolent, and hard to manage. The girl was close to her father emotionally, maybe too close since the two of them regularly sided against Tracy, treating her as an interloper. As is often the case in second marriages, Tracy felt insecure
and believed her husband was more committed to his daughter than to her. As a

consequence, the couple frequently had fierce and ugly battles so that Tracy and her family lived with enormous stress and tension. She felt trapped in her marriage and didn't know how she and her husband were ever going to create a viable family life. Then one morning as she was taking a shower, she found a lump. "When will it ever end?" Tracy asked. "I have little help from my family as I fight for my life."

We talked about the high chronic stress she was experiencing and her need for support as she confronted cancer. Could she and her husband go into marital or family counseling? "My husband refuses," she responded tersely. I tried another tack. Could she leave the situation for a while, go stay with a relative or friend, and just focus on reclaiming her health? "We don't have much extra cash now, and besides I have nowhere to go," she answered.

Feeling blocked and frustrated by her answers, I began to tell her about my situation and to talk about nutrition, explaining that research shows breast cancer responds to an anticancer diet. She listened and agreed that she needed to make significant dietary changes. "But it's hard, because just about every night my husband orders pizza."

Pizza! Knowing I was probably tossing a hand grenade into a smoldering war zone, I quietly asked, "Does your husband want you to survive?"

Silence. Finally, moments later, Tracy said in a voice I strained to hear, "I don't know."

Before we hung up, I urged her to find someone to talk to—her pastor or a counselor—so she would have a trained professional to help her sort through her life and make some important decisions. Because her family consumed so much of her emotional energy, Tracy had few inner resources left for the necessary work of caring for herself. What she needed and did not have was a loving, supportive family and abundant friends as she worked to get well. Instead, she was struggling with angry, difficult people, with no relief in sight.

WE ALL KNOW DIFFICULT PEOPLE

Let's face it. We all have difficult people in our lives. In fact, before ten o'clock this morning, I had two painful conversations, one with a close friend, which was resolved happily, and one with a relative, which left me with a knot in my stomach.

So as I write this, I'm working through hurt feelings from the last exchange while I pray and figure out what to do next.

To be human is to struggle with other humans. In talking with cancer survivors, I have learned that at the time of their diagnosis many had tangled relationships that caused them emotional pain and taxed their limited physical and psychological resources. In *Love and Survival,* Dr. Dean Ornish, one of America's most famous cardiologists, suggests that people who develop cancer have had greater difficulty with their adult relationships than people who are healthy. He cites a survey of men with lung cancer conducted in Scotland in the fifties by Dr. David Kisser and his colleagues. Not only did these men have painful early lives (some had experienced the death of one or both parents), but they "tended to have more disturbed interpersonal relationships" and had a hard time sharing their deepest selves with friends and spouses.[1]

Whatever the specific source, troubled, unresolved, tangled relationships produce great emotional pain and affect our health adversely. Difficult people can create chronic stress, increase our anxiety, engage us in conflicts, reject us, seek to control us, or try to induce guilt. The list goes on and on.

Thus, we need to understand how to resolve difficult relationships in a responsible way to reduce the stress on our already compromised immune systems. It's tough to get well if we are locked in conflict with those closest to us. In fact, one study found that couples who had been married a stunning forty-two years had weakened immune systems if they argued constantly.[2]

But you don't have to have been married for decades to experience a depression of your immune system. In fact, a study of ninety *newly married* couples found that marital conflict depressed their immune systems as well. Dr. Ornish says that our immune systems are simply less effective whenever we fight with our spouses, even if we are otherwise happy in our marriages.[3] He adds that women experience more negative immunological changes as a result of conflict than men.[4] Furthermore, Linda Seligman states in *Promoting a Fighting Spirit* that "people with cancer whose relationships are difficult or unrewarding may have a poor outcome."[5]

Can we rework tangled, painful relationships and turn them around? Some of them. Will they become all we desire them to be? Probably not. Must we reduce our expectations so that we also reduce our emotional pain? Yes. Will it take energy, time, and effort? Absolutely. And it will require honest soul-searching to understand how we contribute to our difficult relationships, and it means that we, as well as these "DPs," will have to modify our behavior.

Now all of this can sound daunting and overwhelming, especially if you have just discovered you have cancer. After all, you have critical treatment decisions to make, and you may elect to have surgery and undergo chemotherapy or radiation. All of this can leave you wiped out for months.

But after you move beyond the initial period of cancer treatment and have recouped some of your emotional and physical energy, that's the time to start working on painful relationships. Especially with those people you live with or see daily.

MAKE A LIST

When you're ready, make a list of the people who have hurt you, both recently and in the past—at least those who readily come to mind. As Harold Bloomfield, M.D., says in *Making Peace with Your Past,* most of the people on the list will be those we love the most. He writes, "One of Freud's most enduring contributions to psychology was the insight that love always contains the seeds of hatred."[6] We need, says Bloomfield, to give ourselves permission to list each person who inspires feelings of anger and hurt without feeling bad or guilty.[7] Then we can methodically begin to work on these relationships, one by one. As we examine each difficult relationship, we need to ask ourselves:

- Why does this relationship cause me pain?
- Is it realistic to assume my needs for love and respect will be met in this relationship, or is this relationship all about the other person? In other words, am I involved with someone who is narcissistic and is using me to meet his or her needs and unwilling or unable to care about mine?
- How open is this person to working on the relationship?
- What do I contribute to the negativity of this relationship, and how should I change my behavior for the better?
- Do I need to set better boundaries?
- Should this relationship even continue?

STOP REPRESSING YOUR FEELINGS

As you examine your troubled relationships with rigor and painful honesty, allow yourself to *feel* what you may have suppressed for years—all the anger, hurt, sadness, resentment, bitterness, even despair.

In *How People Grow,* Dr. Henry Cloud and Dr. John Townsend write, "Anger is a problem-solving emotion designed to protect what is good and valuable."[8] So why do some of us have great difficulty with this emotion? Cloud and Townsend suggest that sometimes we don't express anger about the bad things that happen to us because we learned as children that to do so was dangerous.[9] How many of you still deny your anger at the relative who sexually abused you as a child, or at the friend who betrayed you, or at the spouse who hurt you deeply? Abused children turn their anger inward and blame themselves. Or if we were overwhelmed as children of divorce and badly treated by a divorced parent and a new spouse, we may even as adults feel like vulnerable four-year-olds in their presence. If we feel insecure in a friendship, we may not challenge it, fearing that our friend will walk away. And those locked in troubled marriages sometimes have learned that all the anger gets expressed by only one partner. If your husband or wife has all the anger privileges in your marriage, chances are you have internalized your anger and rage. It's time to stop.

USE ANGER; DON'T LET IT USE YOU

Use anger as a tool to create positive change in your relationships by becoming assertive in expressing how you feel. Make sure your needs are addressed in each important relationship. Strive for reciprocity and mutually satisfying relationships.

We get angry because we have been hurt and the wrong has not been redressed. Sometimes we get depressed because of the smoldering hostility locked inside. As I told a young woman recently who has been treated harshly by her mother, "Stuffing all those angry feelings won't solve your problems. It may even hurt you physiologically. Tell your mother how she has hurt you. Speak clearly and respectfully. Be brave. You are no longer a powerless child."

When we become assertive and calmly tell people how they have hurt us, we feel more powerful, no matter how they respond. Our self-respect increases because we are not allowing others to disrespect us. Sometimes we are fortunate, and the other person listens and says, "I'm sorry I hurt you. Will you forgive me?" Other times the individual can't hear us and refuses to acknowledge any wrong. While the latter is painful, it doesn't hurt us as much as nursing the wrong, stewing about it, or even reacting explosively. Acknowledge your anger, but deal with it constructively.

Recently I had a difficult telephone conversation with my closest female friend. She and I needed to clear the air because we had both said things that hurt the other. At first I got angry and told her so, but then I forced myself to be quiet and hear her out. After I listened, I told her what she had said made sense, and I apologized for giving her occasional heartburn. Then I put my needs on the table. Could she hear what I was saying? She showed me by her response that she heard me. We laughed—our way of defusing tension in our twenty-year friendship. Finally, we agreed to make some changes in the way we relate. Before we hung up, I asked her if she was satisfied with where we were. She said she was, and I told her I felt okay too. And it was only eight o'clock in the morning!

What a lot of work, energy, and commitment had gone into that conversation—for both of us. As I headed for my morning cup of green tea, I was grateful for my friend, because I have learned I can count on her. Although we do not have similar interests (she has been trying to get me to play bridge and golf for years, to no avail), we share twenty years of personal history. Together, we have buried our mothers. I have been present at her children's weddings, and she has come to mine. We also have similar values, one of which is to work through hurt feelings and conflict, because the friendship matters to both of us.

If we don't keep clean slates with our friends and families, then our anger may turn into bitterness and resentment, phantom emotions that take root in our hearts and are hard to ferret out. Over time we even forget how much bitterness and resentment we harbor until we encounter the offending person or God shows us the true nature of our hearts.

DEAL WITH BITTERNESS

One way to deal with bitterness and resentment is to write a letter to the person who has hurt you, even though you may never mail it. As a therapist, I often asked clients to try this exercise. One woman who felt hurt and angry toward her rejecting father brought her letter to therapy to read aloud. In the letter she told her father how much it hurt that he had lavished time and attention on her brother while ignoring her. She had yearned for him to spend time with her, both as a child and as an adult. My client cried as she read the letter, and then we talked about what she wanted to do with it. She chose to modify the letter and send it to her father. To my surprise, her father responded with some degree of understanding and compassion. His life had changed; he had retired from the military, and he finally realized the importance of improving his relationship with his daughter. He asked for her forgiveness and then bought her an airline ticket to Montana, his home. He wanted to repair their relationship, and because she had worked through her anger, my client was ready to go.

I personally have used this technique on several occasions, pouring out my anger, hurt, and frustration on paper within the safety of my home. Later I've thrown these letters away, but they have freed me from toxic emotions that had a stranglehold on my mind.

The Beauty of Forgiveness

No matter how difficult or painful a relationship is, we must ultimately forgive the person who has hurt us or wronged us to give our bodies the best chance to heal. And to have a clear conscience, we must ask those we've offended to forgive us as well.

Forgiving is seldom easy, but it is the only way we will ever be free from the shackles of blame, hurt, and resentment. Dr. Harold Bloomfield says that "when you forgive, the one to whom you give the most is you. You are giving back to yourself the vital life energy that has been consumed by bitterness."[10] Energy. That's something most people need in greater abundance, especially those of us striving to get well.

Also, forgiveness is mandated by Scripture. In Matthew 18, Peter asks Jesus how many times he should forgive his brother, up to seven times perhaps? Jesus gives the stunning reply: "seventy-seven times" (verse 22) or as some translations render it, "seventy times seven" (KJV). Jesus continues by telling his disciples the parable of the unmerciful servant. A master forgives his servant his huge debt, but later the servant refuses to forgive a smaller debt owed him by another servant. Christ concludes with these sobering words:

Then the master called the servant in. "You wicked servant," he said, "I canceled all that debt of yours because you begged me to. Shouldn't you have had mercy on your fellow servant just as I had on you?" In anger his master turned him over to the jailers to be tortured, until he should pay back all he owed.

This is how my heavenly Father will treat each of you unless you forgive your brother from your heart. (verses 32-35)

What powerful words. Scary words. But they underscore just how important God considers forgiveness in human relationships. In *Letters to an American Lady*, the late C. S. Lewis wrote to Mary, a widow four years older than Lewis: "Remember that He has promised to forgive you *as*, and only *as*, you forgive them."[11] Lewis added, "Try not to think—much less, speak—of *their* sins. One's own are a much more profitable theme! And if, on consideration, one can find no faults on one's own side, then cry for mercy; for this *must* be a dangerous delusion."[12]

In another letter Lewis took a somewhat softer stance when discussing the relationship between forgiving and being forgiven. In speaking about the parable of the unjust judge, he wrote, "I...get quite a new feeling about 'If you forgive, you will be forgiven.' I don't believe it is, as it sounds, a bargain. The forgiving and being forgiven are really the very same thing. But one is safe as long as one keeps trying."[13]

As long as one keeps trying. I remember how comforted I was when I read Lewis's words as a Wheaton College student, struggling to forgive my mother. Here was possibly the most famous Christian writer of the twentieth century saying that all we have to do is keep trying to forgive, to put our will in motion even when our emotions scream in rebellion. God seems to honor our simple willingness to forgive, as long as we, in Lewis's words, *keep trying*. The lovely thing is that eventually the emotions do catch up with the will.

Lewis wasn't speaking just theoretically. He had struggled for years to forgive an abusive schoolmaster until finally one day he realized it had happened: Forgiveness had worked its alchemy at the level of his emotions. He wrote to Mary on July 6, 1963:

Do you know, only a few weeks ago I realized suddenly that I at last had forgiven the cruel schoolmaster who so darkened my childhood. I'd been trying to do it for years; and like you, each time I thought I'd done it, I found, after a week or so it all had to be attempted over again. But this time I feel sure it is the real thing. And (like learning to swim or ride a bicycle) the moment it does happen it seems so easy and you wonder why on earth you didn't do it years ago.[14]

Lewis died on November 6, 1963, exactly four months to the day after he wrote these astonishing words. Please don't miss the fact that it took this famous Christian most of his life to finally *feel* that he had forgiven the schoolmaster who had wounded him so deeply. Mercifully, beautifully, our Lord allowed Lewis to understand this was a *fait accompli* mere months before he was ushered into heaven.

LANEY'S STORY

As Lewis showed us, the road to forgiveness can be a long one. One woman I'll call Laney shares how she took the high road and forgave after being hurt deeply.

More than twenty years ago Laney's husband, Ron, a prominent oncologist, left her for another woman. He couldn't have picked a worse time. The previous year Laney's elegant Italian mother had died from lymphoma, a type of cancer that is usually treatable, after only nine months. Laney's grief was short-circuited, however, because she soon learned she was three months pregnant with her fourth child. And when her baby was only six months old and his siblings ages thirteen, twelve, and nine, Laney discovered she had a lump in her breast.

Since she was premenopausal and had a number of malignant nodes, Laney elected to undergo chemotherapy, radiation, and an ovariectomy to decrease the production of estrogen—a painful course of treatment. During her year on chemo, Laney suspected Ron was involved with another woman. "People tried to tell me—subtly—that something was going on, but when I confronted Ron, he only said he wasn't sure of himself or he needed personal space or he felt trapped in the provider role." She added, "He was forty at the time and was probably in the middle of a full-blown midlife crisis. As he talked about all the opportunities that had passed him by, I listened and felt like an old shoe that had serviced someone well."

As Laney was getting into the car to go to the hospital for her mastectomy, her husband started to cry. "You're being so strong; I'm falling apart," he said. So Laney did what she had always done in their long marriage—she encouraged her husband while denying her own need for support and comfort. "Our marriage was all about comforting Ron. I comforted him because his role as an oncologist was to comfort others." Who comforted her? "My comfort came from family and friends. But you need to understand that at that time my husband was my hero. I told myself, 'If I die tomorrow, it's okay. I've been loved.'"

As she was finishing her last round of chemo, Ron moved out. By this time he was deeply involved with a hospice nurse he had met at work. Aware of her existence, Laney asked, "Do you love her?" to which Ron replied, "I don't know. I still love you." The day he left, Laney told Ron angrily that her chances of happiness were greater than his because she was emotionally stronger than he. She also said, with great pain, that she would get to raise their confused, hurt, wonderful children. Ron drove away, and Laney turned back toward the house, their eighteen-month-old son in her arms.

I visited Laney during that terrible time. We had been friends for years, and I was saddened that my wise, lovely friend was locked in the throes of a Greek tragedy. For about a year after Ron left, Laney was clinically depressed. This woman, who had felt all of her life that she was blessed, didn't want to get out of bed in the morning. "I only got up because I could hear my baby crying," she told me. "I didn't want to answer the phone. I pulled the blinds down."

She finally came to herself when her brother, John, a happily married surgeon living in the same city, asked her, "Are you enjoying being depressed?"

Shocked, Laney snapped, "Of course not!" Then John, who had always been emotionally close to his sister, told her in no uncertain terms that she needed to get help.

Laney realized John was right. At some level she did "enjoy" being depressed, and this awareness spurred her to action. Soon she found a psychiatrist who told her, "You're slow to anger, but the truth is, you're very angry. And you have a right to be. Your husband broke an important contract. He promised to love you and your children and provide for your care." Then the psychiatrist encouraged her to confront her husband—to yell and scream if she felt like it.

Laughing, Laney told me that she and a girlfriend drove to Ron's apartment that very afternoon. "Ron was moving in that day, and he actually smiled when he saw me," said Laney, aware of the incongruity of the situation. "He thought I'd come to assist him, to protect his image in the community. When we went into his apartment, he was shocked as I began to yell at the top of my lungs, 'You have nerve! Let *me* tell your neighbors what you have done. You have left your wife and four children for another woman.'"

She sighed and continued her story. "Since this was something I'd never done before, Ron was flabbergasted. But it felt good. Really good. That experience set me free."

During our twice yearly midnight talks, I have noticed that Laney's attitude toward Ron has softened, especially since he was diagnosed with ALS about ten years ago. The majority of those with ALS die within five years, slowly losing their motor capacity, their ability to talk, to eat, and to swallow, until finally only their brains remain vibrant and alive.

Fortunately for Ron, he has a form of ALS that develops slowly. While he has given up his medical practice and moves about in a wheelchair, he is still able to feed himself and talk, though his speech is slurred and hard to understand. Since he and Laney live in the same city, she has seen him, the nurse he married soon after their divorce, and his daughter from the second marriage at all their children's celebrations and special events over the years.

Has she forgiven him? "Yes," she said. "But forgiveness is a process. Some walk it faster than others. When I decided I would no longer be angry at Ron because it was hurting me and my children, that's when I began to forgive him. By then I felt more secure and had substantially rebuilt my life. Now I feel sorry for him because he has this terrible disease and because he has missed out on the lives of four wonderful children." She continued, "While I've let go of the anger, it's like a scar. I don't look at it or even see it, but it's part of my past."

She then reflected on the irony of her current situation. Ron left her when she had breast cancer because he was afraid she was going to die, and he wanted to be free of marital and parental constraints. Yet today Laney is the one who is free, teaching her beloved third graders, traveling with her girlfriends—the "four musketeers"—to near and distant places, and spending her summers at a lakeside cottage with family and friends. Ron, on the other hand, spends his days in a wheelchair. In thinking about this reversal of fortune, Laney said fiercely, "When I look at Ron, I don't believe his ALS is 'just deserts' as some people have indicated. I can't believe God punished him for leaving our marriage and betraying me by giving him this disease. But this outcome is not what either of us expected years ago."

Laney had a recurrence of breast cancer several years ago, but she is philosophical about life after cancer. She knows she has survived longer than most, and she fully understands that life is chancy at best. "We can't ever take tomorrow for granted. I'm happy that I'm alive and that I have people around me I count on and who count on me. I have a wonderful, dependable brother and an angel for a sister-in-law and four great children. When you know you're loved, that brings a certain sense of peace and security."

Indeed. At the end of our conversation, Laney paused and quietly summed up the last twenty-two years of her life: "Who knows but that cancer was a blessing in disguise."

Let Go of Toxic Relationships

Even though to be truly free we must forgive those who have hurt us, sometimes we also have to end toxic relationships. What do I mean by a toxic relationship? The woman who is married to an abusive husband who refuses to change, or the man who is yoked to a serial adulteress will find it difficult to stay in a destructive relationship and hope to recover from cancer. The Bible, which draws a hard line on divorce, does allow it on grounds of adultery. And I have heard several pastors advocate separation in instances of physical abuse or incest.

I am no advocate of divorce, having gone through a painful, unwanted divorce at age twenty-nine. Nor do I believe adultery necessitates divorce. But I also don't believe that any marriage is worth dying for. If a marriage is utterly toxic and destructive, and the spouse is unrepentant and unwilling to change or get help, it is better to separate for a while and concentrate on getting well. It takes abundant energy to work on restoring a troubled marriage. When I worked as a therapist, I first helped my clients recover from their depression before suggesting we invite their spouses in for joint sessions. The same principle applies with serious illness. First, concentrate on getting well. Then work on the marriage if it can be saved.

Dr. Gonzalez told me about one of his patients who came with diagnosed prostate cancer. Both husband and wife came for the initial visit, and then the wife proceeded to rail at her husband in front of Gonzalez, a virtual stranger. Why? According to Gonzalez, her accomplished husband was not, in her estimation, good enough. He simply didn't measure up as a human being. At the end of the visit, Gonzalez asked to see the man alone at the next appointment, at which time Gonzalez told him that if he wanted to have a fighting chance at getting well, he had to deal with his toxic marriage.[15]

Sometimes the toxic relationship is not with a spouse but with a friend or relative who is narcissistic ("it's all about me") and wounding. In that instance, imagine that you are taking a restorative, open-ended sabbatical and gently drift away. At the very least, limit contact, or have a third party present to limit the negativity. It may possibly be months or years before the two of you are genuinely reconciled and the relationship has changed and become healthier. In any event, you have only so much energy and time. Cancer, as one woman said, is a "now" disease. *Now* is the time to concentrate your energies on getting well rather than on relationships that pull you down and are poisonous to your very soul. Do what you can in your own heart—forgive, seek forgiveness, restore what can be restored— but don't hang on to destructive relationships.

RELEASE THE PERSON TO GOD

When we have done all we can to work through our difficult relationships and to forgive and ask for forgiveness, it is then time to release these people to God. We are no longer bound through our anger or resentment to the person who hurt us. Nor is he or she bound to us. And even if the other person refuses to forgive us or to work toward a healthier relationship, we can be inwardly free. Except for continuing to pray for the other person, our soul's work is done.

Perhaps at a later time God will engineer the miracle of restoration in our most broken relationships. We can hope. We can pray. But as we wait, we can live our days in peace and joy. We can finally be free in our hearts and minds, and receive the immeasurable benefit to our souls and bodies.

EMBRACING LIFE

Hold fast to dreams, for if dreams die,
Life is a broken winged bird that cannot fly.
LANGSTON HUGHES

The more connected you are to life, the healthier you are.
JAMES LYNCH

For fourteen years I have had to force myself to go to work each day," said the attractively dressed, thirty-something redhead sitting across from me. "My first corporate job was the worst. Every morning I would lie in bed and fantasize about calling in sick. But I couldn't, so I would drag myself off to work. Some days the hours, even the minutes, just dragged by. After several years I got a much better job at a new company, with a lot more money. But it's still the same. The truth is, I really hate corporate life. It's not who I am at all. Each time I take a new job, I feel as if I have the chance to get out, and then I end up betraying myself again. I feel like the most spineless person, and I hate myself for it. I worry that I'll never pursue my dream to be a writer and that I'll end up alone with a lot of great clothes and nothing else to show for all these years. It will all have been wasted."

In the stillness of my office we talked about Olivia's ten-year battle with insomnia, chronic fatigue, and anxiety. More life coach than therapist, I asked her what kept her from taking a sabbatical to write a novel and break into magazine writing. One by one, we removed the roadblocks in her path. She decided to talk to her employer about going part time and to use savings to bridge the gap for the six months or more it would take to finish her novel.

As she turned to leave, she thanked me. "I need to feel like there are possibilities. When I think about another twenty years of this, I lose hope. But now I feel as though in pursuing my dream I am giving myself a gift—the gift of believing in myself."

As she left my office that day, I thought of where I had been six years ago. I, too, felt trapped in a life that didn't fit. I also had insomnia, apathy, little joy, and a profound lack of energy. But I didn't know what kind of new life I wanted, and I was clueless about how to make the necessary changes so my spirit could soar. Then along came cancer, the premier wake-up call. Suddenly I knew that if I didn't create a life that worked for me, a life with less stress and more possibilities, I might not survive. But how to begin?

When I discovered *Cancer As a Turning Point,* by Dr. Lawrence LeShan, the book gave me a whole new way of looking at my life, cancer, and the future. LeShan states in his book that when he first started working with cancer patients decades ago, he used a traditional psychotherapeutic approach: He focused on what was *wrong* with the person. How did he or she become this way? What could be done about it?[1] Unfortunately, few of his patients survived. LeShan determined that focusing on the negative didn't make sense when the people in front of him were desperately ill, scared, and overwhelmed by the side effects of their treatment.

That's when he created a new therapeutic approach. LeShan began to focus on what was *right* with the person in front of him—the individual's special and unique ways of being, relating, and creating. In working with a cancer patient, he asked, "What is his special music to beat out in life, his unique song to sing so that when he is singing it he is glad to get up in the morning and glad to go to bed at night?" LeShan wanted to know what would give his patients zest, enthusiasm, and a feeling of deep involvement with their lives.[2]

He found that the cancer patients he worked with had, at the unconscious level, ceased to believe they could ever create the lives they yearned for or have the quality of relationships they so desired. He theorized that this lack of aliveness and joy depressed their immune systems and made them vulnerable to cancer. His task: to help them mobilize their immune systems by discovering what made them feel fully alive and excited about life. LeShan puts it this way: "The therapist has to lead the patient to give up fears and anxieties, concerns about 'success' and the opinions of others, and ultimately become concerned about his or her authentic development."[3] While LeShan believes that understanding one's past and the patterns that have contributed to cancer is important, he realizes that patients need to change their lives immediately if they are to survive.

Too Busy for Cancer

LeShan tells the story of Carol, a successful vice president of a large firm in her late thirties, whose doctor told her that the large black moles on her back were indeed malignant. She showed up in LeShan's office soon thereafter, and together they began to explore her life. She told LeShan that she hated her job, that she struggled with self-loathing because she wasn't married, and that the only job she had ever been excited about was working with physically handicapped adults when she was in college. As a result of their conversations—and to the chagrin of her parents and siblings—Carol sold her penthouse, quit her job, and enrolled in a graduate program in special education. She loved it.

In the meantime, what was happening to the moles? At first the black melanoma moles seemed to increase in size, but after a few months they stopped growing. At the six-month mark, the angry moles began to shrink until soon they were no longer visible.

Ten years after Carol completed her therapy she ran into LeShan one day. She asked him, "Do you know why I've never gotten in touch with you?" When the psychologist shook his head, she replied, "It's because I've been too busy living my life to have time for any such nonsense as cancer, psychotherapy, or you."

Instead of being offended by her remarks, LeShan writes, "For a psychotherapist that was a combination of the Congressional Medal of Honor and the Nobel Prize."[4] When LeShan saw her a second time, several years later, she had left special ed to run a charitable foundation, but she told him she was still happy and fulfilled. She had created a life that gave her zest, the opportunity to sing her special song, and the most priceless gift—vibrant health.

The Magic Question

Dr. Gary Cobb, a clinical psychologist trained in behavioral medicine at Brown University who has worked with cancer patients since the eighties, echoes LeShan's perspective and works with his cancer patients to help them embrace life. He is quick to admit, however, that this is no easy task.

According to Cobb, "Many cancer patients have been abandoned by a parent, either physically or emotionally. Their parents may have neglected them or had addiction problems or mental problems. So the cancer patient has great unmet needs. This breeds a deep sense of loneliness and the conviction that identity, as well as meaning and purpose, comes from taking care of others." Then the genial psychologist told me, "The cancer patients I've worked with believe they are not really entitled to receive nurture, either self-care or care from others. It's embarrassing for them to receive care since they didn't internalize self-worth, self-respect, self-dignity as children." He continued, "They tend to be worriers, rescuers, caretakers who are conscientious and hard working; in fact, they tend to take responsibility for the whole world. And this sense of responsibility weighs on them and hurts their health."

Another reason cancer patients find it hard to embrace life, says Cobb, is their very legitimate fear of death. "They don't know if the things they are doing will help them survive or if the medical community can assure them they will be safe. Most people assume cancer is a death sentence, and some say, 'Now that I've been diagnosed with cancer, of course I'm going to die from this disease.'" Because of this, Cobb believes that many begin to make a subtle but real psychological adjustment to cancer and unconsciously prepare to die. He adds, "A 40 percent chance of survival, for most people, gets translated into a 60 percent chance of death. Instead of embracing life and enjoying the time they have left, many resign themselves to the disease. They tell me, 'What if I put out all this effort and don't make it?'" Cobb believes that when cancer patients prepare for their own deaths, it weakens their immune systems, thereby creating a greater likelihood of dying prematurely. "Although you have a disease that could kill you, this doesn't mean you should embrace the inevitability of your own death," says this psychologist, who had a heart attack a year ago and truly understands a brush with one's mortality.

While Cobb respects the fear many of his cancer patients feel, he tells them, "It is possible the disease will kill you, but it is also possible it won't. So what happens if you're forty-five years old when you're diagnosed with cancer, and you live until you're ninety-five, and you've spent the last fifty years of your life preparing for a death that didn't occur? Will you then realize you've lost fifty years?" Cobb believes those with cancer should make a conscious effort to say, "The sun is up, I'm still kicking, and I'm going to live the best life I can."

How does Dr. Cobb help his patients choose life? "I use an old therapeutic technique called the magic question," he told me. "Basically, I ask the person with cancer to paint a picture of his ideal life, the life he would live if he had sufficient time, resources, and energy. If he didn't have cancer, how would he choose to live?"

Recognizing that some don't believe they will live long enough to fulfill their dreams, Cobb tells them, "It's possible you might not live long enough to realize your ideal life, but it is also possible you may. However, if you're not dedicating yourself to that goal, I guarantee you'll never live the life of your dreams, no matter how long you live."

He adds: "If you shoot for the moon and you get only halfway there, that's pretty good. Lots of people have goals and aspirations that they may or may not achieve, but it's not the final destination that's valuable. It's the motivation, the drive, the incentive to get up every morning because you have this goal that creates meaning and purpose in your life."

COMMIT TO YOURSELF

According to Cobb, those who are able to embrace life commit to doing a personal inventory and determine what's really important to them. They let go of peripheral concerns and refocus their energies and priorities. Sometimes they make vocational changes; sometimes they elect to stay with their jobs and excel in that arena. Others try to deepen their intimate relationships. Cobb says, "Often they stop worrying about income or whether they have a great house or how the kids will go to college. Instead, they begin to appreciate and value each new day, learning to have faith that everything essential will be provided.

"Basically, when people who have cancer embrace life, they are choosing to escalate their value to the level of everyone else's," says Cobb.[5]

What would make you feel fully alive in every cell of your body? What would make you want to leap out of bed in the morning and embrace the day? Are you doing what you love to do each day? Or are you trapped in a profession or lifestyle that wears you down, saps your energy, and dampens your spirit? Like several people in a previous chapter, do you feel trapped in a cage? How can you redesign your life to make it more joyful?

As you consider what brings you joy, look beyond the boundaries of your current life. Ephesians 2:10 says, "For we are God's workmanship, created in Christ Jesus to do good works, which God prepared in advance for us to do." What are these good works? They generally involve service to others who can't pay us back—the sick, the poor, the powerless. This is what gives our lives meaning and joy. I have a framed quote by Dr. Albert Schweitzer that states: "The only ones among us who will be truly happy are those who have sought and found how to serve."

One person who has done this is Geri Blair, an African American woman who found a lump in her breast in 1985 and was still alive and going strong thirteen years later. Because she had lost a mother, two sisters, one niece, and an aunt to this disease, she immediately had the lump biopsied. It proved malignant, and she had surgery and chemotherapy to treat her cancer. When she landed back in the hospital with a staph infection, Geri believed she was dying and that only God could help her. She writes: "I promised God that if He healed my body of the infection, I would dedicate my life to Him."[6]

When Geri got well, she was amazed to learn about the high mortality rate among African American women who acquire breast cancer. In 1992, she cofounded Minority Women with Breast Cancer to educate others about this disease. She had no money, only faith. Over the years she and her cofounder have taken the University of Cleveland's mobile mammography van into minority neighborhoods, provided free prostheses for women who couldn't afford them, and worked with pastors to encourage them to speak to their congregations about the need for breast-cancer screening.

This woman runs a hundred-person support group each month, speaks frequently, and has been a peer reviewer for breast-cancer research funding in Washington, D.C., but she also finds time to talk to women one-on-one about breast cancer. She writes, "Do I get tired? No! I am doing the work that the Lord wants me to do. It is my promise to Him and I am enjoying it immensely every day."[7]

Hold Fast to Dreams

For most of my life I have had outrageous dreams, like publishing books, getting a doctorate, living abroad, and having a second chance at a loving, committed marriage. These were big dreams for a small-town girl who was the first person in my extended family to finish college. Growing up in extreme poverty, my mother and I lived in rooming houses or, at best, a three-room apartment. Mother worked hard at women's dress shops or as a telephone operator but never made more than minimum wage. We couldn't afford a car, television set, or air conditioning, and since mother couldn't feed and clothe us simultaneously, she decided we would dress well and stay slim. I had no reason to hope for a life beyond my small town. But I dreamed otherwise.

In ninth grade I signed up for the college prep course rather than the secretarial track, not because I thought the latter demeaning but because I had absolutely no talent or interest in that area. Education was my ticket out of poverty. God provided, giving me wonderful benefactors to help pay my way through Wheaton College—a local surgeon, the owner of a factory where I folded baby clothes one summer during college, and at the end of my four years, S. S. Kresge, the owner of the chain that later became K-Mart.

Years later, when I found myself in the midst of a painful, unwanted divorce, the Lord enabled me to realize a lifelong dream of European travel. My Aunt Stella took my daughters and me to Germany, France, and Switzerland. In addition, with modest child support I was able to live in England for two years as part of a vibrant L'Abri Christian community. My friends at L'Abri provided emotional support and spiritual encouragement as I rebuilt my life. Then in 1978 I published my first book and later obtained my doctorate, with Don's encouragement and practical help.

But in my early fifties, I stopped dreaming. I became a "broken-winged bird" that could not fly. Basically, I lost my sense of a fulfilling future. In time, I developed cancer.

As God and I have worked together to heal and renew my mind, body, and spirit, gratefully, I have begun to dream again. But my dreams are different now. I no longer dream of achievement or about globetrotting. Instead I dream of owning a grandmother's house close to my sweet grandchildren so I can be part of their young lives, of working in integrative medicine as a psychologist, of savoring the seasons with Don in our mountain perch. Mostly I dream of being useful to God, and I stand on tiptoe, waiting to see what direction he will steer my life.

What about you? Have you held fast to immune-enhancing dreams? If not, could you dream again and envision "a future and a hope"? No matter how sick you feel, can you get alone and ask yourself the "magic question": "If I didn't have cancer, what would I want to do with the rest of my life?" Get ready—you may find that you begin to live a life that exceeds your wildest imaginings.

My Favorite Embracing-Life Story

Dr. Lawrence LeShan writes of Ethel, a woman who had metastasized breast cancer and was sent home to die. Frightened and upset, Ethel began seeing a psychiatrist, Dr. Joost A. M. Meerloo, to discover how best to live the rest of her life. During their conversations, she told Dr. Meerloo that all of her life she had wanted to travel on an ocean liner but caring for her home and family had prevented it. She loved the sea and laughingly said that being a sailor would have been ideal for her had her gender been different.

Meerloo pointed out that since her husband was dead and her children were grown, why not travel now? Even though her oncologist had given her only a couple of months to live and she was afraid she would die at sea, Dr. Meerloo encouraged her to embrace life by saying, "With the sickness you have, what could happen to you on the water that couldn't happen on land?"

Finally convinced, Ethel invested her entire savings in a first-class cabin on the *Queen Mary*, which was circling the globe at that time. LeShan writes, "Four months later she stormed into Meerloo's office and berated him, saying, 'Here I've spent all my money. I'm broke and I'm still alive.'"[8]

When Dr. Meerloo asked Ethel if she would have preferred the alternative, they burst out laughing. Since she relished life at sea, Meerloo helped her secure a job on a Holland America cruise ship, working in a boutique. Eight years later Ethel was still alive, and every Christmas she sent her psychiatrist a Christmas card, telling him how utterly fulfilling her new life was.[9] She kept sending him cards… until he died.

She loved her life and felt it was completely fulfilling. In having the courage to embrace life and live her dream, Ethel outlived both her oncologist's prognosis and her psychiatrist. No small feat for a woman given just two months to live.

Whether we live one year or forty after cancer, what matters most is the quality of our lives, the lovingkindness of our relationships, and the luminosity of our souls. Our days here are numbered, always have been and always will be. In fact, Psalm 139 says they were numbered in heaven before the dances of our lives began. And when our days are used up, we will vanish from this earth like the mist that rises from my mountain every morning.

What will you do with the only day you can claim for sure—today? How will you embrace your life this next hour? This is my prayer for you:

May the Lord bless you and keep you all the days of your life,
and may you find and live the life for which you were born.

STRENGTHENING

THE SPIRIT

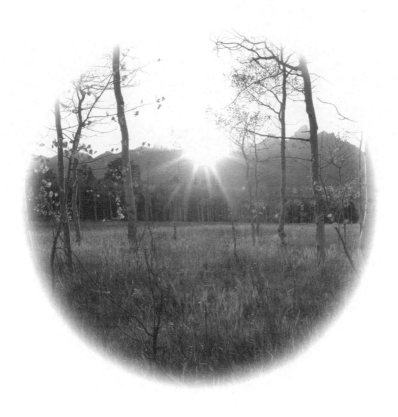

THE HEALING POWER
OF FAITH

I have heard your prayer and seen your tears; I will heal you.

2 KINGS 20:5

Faith is to believe what we do not see: the reward of this faith is to see what we believe.

ST. AUGUSTINE

Six years ago I stood in the center aisle at Truro Episcopal Church in Fairfax, Virginia, waiting for my turn at the altar rail while I listened to the soft, indistinct voices of clergy and laypeople as they prayed with intensity over the bowed heads of the suppliants at the rail. I felt my husband's warm hands resting on my shoulders as he stood behind me, waiting to accompany me to the front of the church. We had come to this healing conference because I had cancer, and I wanted to have others pray that God would heal me.

Cannon Glennon, a tall man in his sixties with a kind, wrinkled face, was the main speaker that night. He had traveled to the United States from Sydney, Australia, to proclaim to his hungry audience that "our healing is within us." Moved by his words, I awaited my turn to receive prayer for physical and emotional healing. As we waited, I looked around and saw a well-dressed, thirty-something mother holding her baby. She was crying quietly as her husband stood by her side, his arm around her waist. Although her child looked healthy to me, something was obviously wrong. Heartbreakingly wrong. Moments later Glennon bent over the sweet little baby, praying intently. I turned my gaze to a man whose neck was swathed in bandages, an ineffective attempt to conceal a grapefruit-size tumor.

Repelled, I reminded myself that although his cancer was visible, mine was just as real. Several people were in wheelchairs, slowly moving down the three aisles of the grand old church.

Suddenly I became aware of a soft breeze blowing, lifting the gauzy curtains at the partially open windows. *Are you here, Lord?* It crossed my mind that the cool breeze was but a metaphor for the presence of the refreshing, healing Spirit of God.

Glancing to my left, I saw the bowed heads of our dear friends Bill and Sandi Eckert, who had come to pray for us. Feelings of gratitude washed over me as I remembered that the Lord had sent numerous people across my path to comfort and instruct. Then it hit me. While I had sat in pews across the years, watching other people line up for prayer, seldom had I been among them.

Now I was a member of that vast throng of suffering humanity. A beggar with empty hands, standing in need of prayer. And then the thought came, *Why shouldn't I be?*

Pain Happens to All of Us

When trials come, whether physical or psychological, we join the congregation of men and women struggling to make sense out of what's happening to us. As Dr. David Jeremiah, senior pastor of Shadow Mountain Community Church and host of the radio program *Turning Point,* says, "We are either in the midst of a storm, coming out of a storm, or getting ready to go into a storm."[1]

Dr. Jeremiah knows what he's talking about. In 1994 he was diagnosed with aggressive large-cell, non-Hodgkin's lymphoma. His cancer was treated, went into remission, and then in 1998 returned, requiring a stem-cell transplant. When his cancer recurred, Jeremiah told Dr. James Dobson on *Focus on the Family* radio that he struggled intensely and asked God, "Why has this been allowed to return?" He admitted that he came as close as he ever had to what Dobson called the "betrayal barrier"—"that point where you feel God has turned his back on you." However, he emerged from this painful time with a deeper sense of God's love and presence.

Jeremiah says he has no doubt that God has a plan for his life and sees the bigger picture. He also believes having cancer has had its benefits—deepening his compassion for others and making his relationship with the Lord stronger than ever. He adds, "All I have preached for years I have found to be true."[2]

Why was a man who loves God and has served him for years afflicted with this life-threatening disease—twice? Jeremiah was asked this very question when he was at the famed Scripps Clinic in California for his stem-cell transplant. He had been invited, along with his oncologist's rabbi, to speak at the clinic on the topic of faith and cancer. When this question was posed, Jeremiah responded, "There's only one reason. I am human." Later, in his interview with Dobson, Jeremiah stated, "We are a diseased people. Whether we're Christians or non-Christians, cancer touches us alike. There's no free pass when you become a believer." He added, "Pain happens to all of us."

Like others of us who have had cancer, Jeremiah knows his future is uncertain. He told Dobson, "I have no guarantee even now...that I am cancer free. I mean, I could go home tomorrow and find out that it has returned. I live in the reality that this disease is part of my life. Whether it's cured or not, it will always be part of my life; it's like background noise. If I have an unexpected pain or something happens to my system, all the questions come back."[3]

Even though he lives with this terrible uncertainty (worsened because of the cancer's recurrence), Jeremiah said, "I know and I choose to believe in the goodness of God, in spite of things that happen that would make anyone question."[4] Folks, that's faith in operation. The kind of sturdy, heroic faith that pleases God and serves as a beacon to the rest of us during our moments of suffering and darkness.

THE FAITH FACTOR

The Bible is clear. Faith in a wise, loving God is the hallmark of the believer. Yet what is this thing called faith? Hebrews 11:1 defines it by saying: "Now faith is being sure of what we hope for and certain of what we do not see." This "faith chapter" goes on to chronicle the exploits that men and women in the Bible accomplished because of their faith in an infinite, personal God—people like Abel, Enoch, Noah, Abraham, Isaac, Jacob, Joseph, Moses, and the prostitute Rahab. These were all commended by the writer of Hebrews for their faith, along with the nameless ones who were stoned, chained, flogged, sawed in two, and put to death by the sword. The biblical view suggests that faith in God is not for the weak-kneed or fainthearted. Nor does our faith guarantee us an easy ride to heaven.

Rather, we are told that our faith, which is "more precious than gold," will be honed in the furnace of affliction, deprivation, and pain (see 1 Peter 1:7, KJV).

While we may shrink from the trials that define our character and refine our belief in God's goodness, faith is important to God for reasons we humans have trouble grasping. The Bible reminds us: "Without faith it is impossible to please God, because anyone who comes to him must believe that he exists and that he rewards those who earnestly seek him" (Hebrews 11:6).

Yet cancer and its recurrence severely test our faith, causing us to wonder, sometimes in the middle of the night or just before dawn, if God is punishing us or if he has abandoned us. Does he *really* see our tears, hear our hearts' utterances, care about our souls?

Psychiatrist Harold Koenig, director of Duke University's Center for the Study of Religion/Spirituality and Health, understands the heart's cry when disaster strikes. He told me, "When people get sick, especially with cancer, they usually ask, 'Why me? Why cancer? Why now?' Later, it's 'Why doesn't God heal me? Why hasn't he answered my prayers? Doesn't God love me?' "[5]

Koenig said these are normal reactions to serious illness. "But," he added, "it's important that people not stay there. Studies show that those who stay angry at God or feel he's punishing them are more likely to die over a two-year period."[6] He continued, "But you can't just tell them God is not punishing them. They need to explore their feelings in a safe place, with a chaplain or pastor or priest." According to Koenig, the ultimate goal for the cancer patient is to be able to say, "I've got this disease, but God still loves me. Things will be okay because God is in control."

FAITH MAKES A MEASURABLE DIFFERENCE

Not only is faith in a loving God psychologically and spiritually comforting, but it has profound physiological consequences as well. Faith makes a measurable difference in terms of health, longevity, and quality of life. In his book *The Healing Power of Faith,* Dr. Koenig writes that "hundreds of major studies show that individuals who read the Bible, attend church regularly, pray, and have a vital faith in a loving Creator have significantly lower diastolic blood pressure than those who are less religious."[7] They are hospitalized less often, are less likely to suffer from depression, have stronger immune systems, and live longer than their nonreligious counterparts. Faith also protects against cardiovascular disease and cancer.

And if those with a strong faith in God do get sick, research shows that they, on average, have better medical outcomes than those with little or no religious faith.[8] In fact, Koenig states that the risk of dying from all causes decreases 35 percent for those who attend religious services one or more times per week. One study found that those who attended church more than once a week lived seven years longer than nonattenders. For African Americans, church attendance had an even greater effect, extending their lives by fourteen years.[9] The faith factor matters. Greatly.

THOSE WHO TRUSTED GOD

While research findings can be encouraging and informative, when I was ill, I was more intrigued by what scientists call anecdotal evidence—individuals' stories. I wanted to hear from people who had been on the front lines with disease, those "foot soldiers" who had lived to tell about it. I particularly wanted to hear from those who felt that God had heard their cries and responded with healing in his wings. Fortunately, such stories abound.

Shirley's Story

My friend Shirley Blackman also understands the power of divine intervention. Twenty-six years ago Shirley made two discoveries in rapid succession—that her husband and the father of her four children was having an affair and that she had breast cancer, which had metastasized to six lymph nodes. Soon she was divorced, depressed, and worried about how she was going to rear Craig, the youngest child, alone. Shirley listened intently as her doctor explained that while he would not prescribe chemo (it was too new on the market), he would check her every month for the foreseeable future.

Was Shirley terrified that she had cancer? "I was numb," she told me. "At first I just wanted to get through it—the radical mastectomy and all. I had lots of people praying for me and lots of support from friends and my three grown children. But I wasn't really scared, and I never thought I'd die."

Today this vital eighty-year-old, who told me she feels twenty-five, says her faith is richer, deeper, and stronger than it was years ago when she went through divorce and cancer. Shirley said, "I've learned that nothing happens to you that doesn't first pass by God's eyes. Things that happen he allows, but he's there with you. I had confidence he was taking care of me, and consequently, my faith has only grown stronger over the years. When trials come, we either fall apart or get stronger." Shirley added, "Of course, there are times I get anxious, like right before my yearly mammogram, so I recite 'Trust in the Lord' every five minutes."

Currently Shirley lives a more active life than many who are years younger. Semiretired from nursing, she is involved in a prison ministry, a weekly prayer group, and another small-group fellowship, and every Wednesday night she drives to her church to help with the midweek meal or to attend a missions committee meeting. In addition, she works two days a week at an adult day-care center, caring for those who are older and younger than she. Shirley also makes a weekly trek to the local elementary school to read aloud to first graders. Since Reach for Recovery, a program for women recovering from breast-cancer surgery, was an important adjunct to her own healing process, Shirley periodically drives to a local hospital to tell women who have just had mastectomies that they, too, can get well. Her words, her demeanor, her whole life broadcast a steady, hopeful message: "Look at me. I'm alive and well. You can make it."

When I learned that I had joined the breast-cancer sorority, Shirley was one of the first people I called for support and encouragement. Her calm, soothing voice came over the wire. "Can you trust God with this disease? Can you put your life in his hands and believe that he can and will heal you?" Shirley continues to inspire me today, as she gives new meaning to the words *optimistic* and *resilient*. The past few years have been emotionally wrenching for her as she has watched one daughter go through divorce and another, who lives only a few houses away, discover that she, too, has breast cancer. In addition, in the past three years Shirley has experienced the deaths of her ninety-six-year-old mother, her former husband, and her only sister. Yet Shirley is more than a mere survivor; she is fully alive. She regularly packs her bungalow with friends and family and relishes time with friends, family, and her nine grandchildren. With her genes and her deep faith in a God who loves her, this woman just might make it to a hundred. And then will she feel thirty-five?

Bud and Emily's Story

Have you ever met someone near death who believed that whether he lived or died, he was a winner? Bud Mitchell, an Asheville native who's on the brink of eighty, felt this way over twenty years ago when his doctors gave him a whopping 2 percent chance of surviving liver cancer. Hospitalized for an adverse reaction to chemo, feeling sick and depleted, he prayed to his heavenly Father, "Lord, are you going to take me home to heaven, or are you going to take me home to Bevlyn Drive?" He wasn't scared; he felt he was prepared to die. "I figured it was win-win," said this man who continued to work half-days during his recovery. When he asked his surgeon, the genial Dr. Reavis Eubanks, if he would survive, Eubanks replied, "Absolutely. You've got too many people praying for you." And so he did. "I had prayer like you wouldn't believe," Bud told me.

Bud said he looked at his life and did a mental inventory. "I had a good marriage to a woman who is as near an angel as you can get in this world, and I had so many people praying for me. I figured my only problem was to get well, and that was between me and the Lord." In addition to his win-win attitude and deep faith in God, Bud had two rounds of chemo, surgery to remove the cancerous part of his liver, and three months of daily intake of vitamin C (6,000 units).

At the same time he was struggling with liver cancer, his wife, Emily, discovered she had breast cancer. With an attitude similar to her husband's, Emily, who was a Bible teacher for years, said, "I knew I was not going to die until the Lord was ready for me, and I was not going to get well if he wanted me in heaven. I told my doctor, 'If this thing comes back, don't tell me I'm dying with cancer. I'm living with it until I die. Either way I want to glorify God.'" Emily believes the key to her long survival is her deep faith and her surrender to God's will for her life. "I'm in the Lord's hands, and I'm not going to worry about death," she told me.

At that point Bud, who had listened attentively to his wife, spoke up. "If you're going to worry about death, get prepared to die."

As I left Bud and Emily's house that night, I was buoyed by the radiant faith these two people emanate. Their trust in God has enabled them to deal with cancer and possible death without a lot of worry and anxiety. And years after their diagnoses, they are vital and still alive, testimony to the healing power of faith and the comfort a strong marriage can provide, even in the face of two simultaneous cancer diagnoses!

STRENGTHENING YOUR FAITH

While positive statistics encourage and survivors' stories inspire, at some point the realization dawns: This is my cancer battle. No one can fight it for me. No friend or loved one is going to be wheeled into surgery with me or take the radiation treatments for me. Will God help me? Will he be there for me? Then we begin to grapple with what we truly believe about God and his willingness to heal us. In my own "dark night of the soul," I felt I had two tools for communicating with God: the Bible and prayer. So I picked up my Bible and read it hungrily, and I prayed as I rarely had before.

I ranged through Scripture, dialoging with God and writing down every comforting verse I found, like Isaiah 57:18-19: "I have seen his ways, but I will heal him; I will guide him and restore comfort to him, creating praise on the lips of the mourners in Israel." I was surprised at the plethora of verses on healing, health, and well-being. For example, protection from disease is presented in the Old Testament book of Exodus as the result of obedience to the voice of the Lord: "If you listen carefully to the voice of the LORD your God and do what is right in his eyes, if you pay attention to his commands and keep all his decrees, I will not bring on you any of the diseases I brought on the Egyptians, for I am the LORD, who heals you" (15:26).

Dr. Rex Russell, an invasive radiologist who wrote the excellent book *What the Bible Says About Healthy Living,* comments on this passage: "Considering all the sickness and disease we experience today, could it be that we have not listened carefully enough to the voice of the Lord as related in Exodus 15:26?"[10] According to Russell, who studied both biblical and scientific laws to fully understand the maintenance and recovery of health, *"a large portion of the Scripture focuses on commands, ordinances and statutes that show us how to live on this carefully designed earth."*[11]

In addition, worship of the Lord is connected with a long life span: "Worship the LORD your God, and his blessing will be on your food and water. I will take away sickness from among you…. I will give you a full life span" (Exodus 23:25-26).

When I turned to the Old Testament, I did not encounter a distant, disinterested deity but a God who heals the sick and the brokenhearted. "Praise the LORD, O my soul,…who forgives all your sins and heals all your diseases" (Psalm

103:2-3). He proclaims, "I will restore you to health and heal your wounds" (Jeremiah 30:17). This same heavenly Father "sent forth his word and healed them; he rescued them from the grave" (Psalm 107:20).

In the Gospels I rediscovered that Jesus loved to heal. He healed the blind, the lepers, the boy with evil spirits. He raised the dead—the widow's son, Jairus's daughter, and his friend Lazarus. As he healed, he did so with empathy and compassion. When a leper came to Christ, Jesus was "filled with compassion" as he reached out, touched this societal pariah, and made him clean (Mark 1:40-41). As he encountered a widow crying because her only son had died, "his heart went out to her and he said, 'Don't cry'" (Luke 7:13).

Jesus, who had the power and authority to cast out demons, heal the sick, and raise the dead, also helps us with our fear of death. Hebrews says that Jesus became human and died so that by his death he could destroy the devil, "who holds the power of death," and thereby set us free from the fear of death, which holds us as its slaves (2:14-15). For those of us who live in fear of death or cancer's recurrence, this is good news indeed.

Healing Prayer

While Father and Son love to heal, and that healing is available to us today, the Bible encourages us to pray and ask God for what we need. Christ taught that we are to ask, seek, and knock and do this with persistence. In the book of James, we are directed to pray "the prayer of faith":

> Is any one of you in trouble? He should pray. Is anyone happy? Let him sing songs of praise. Is any one of you sick? He should call the elders of the church to pray over him and anoint him with oil in the name of the Lord. And the prayer offered in faith will make the sick person well; the Lord will raise him up. If he has sinned, he will be forgiven. Therefore confess your sins to each other and pray for each other so that you may be healed. The prayer of a righteous man is powerful and effective. (5:13-16)

King Hezekiah's Story

One famous Old Testament king prayed fervently that God would spare his life, and God granted his request. In Isaiah 38 Hezekiah, who had been king of Judah for fourteen years, became deathly ill. The prophet Isaiah went to him and said, "This is what the LORD says: Put your house in order, because you are going to die; you will not recover" (verse 1). Such ominous words, and coming directly from God through his prophet! What did the king do? The Bible says he "turned his face to the wall and prayed to the LORD, 'Remember, O LORD, how I have walked before you faithfully and with wholehearted devotion and have done what is good in your eyes'" (verses 2-3). And then the good king wept bitterly.

Did the king influence God with his prayer? Yes, because God told Isaiah to turn around and go back to the king with this new message: "I have heard your prayer and seen your tears; I will add fifteen years to your life" (verse 5). In addition, God promised to end Hezekiah's period of chronic stress by defeating the Assyrians who had toppled kingdoms and laid siege to Jerusalem. In fact, 2 Kings 19:35 says that the angel of the Lord killed 185,000 men in the Assyrian camp in the darkness of night.

When I first read this passage years ago, it seemed to me that Hezekiah actually changed God's mind when he prayed. But Jay Richard Love, senior pastor of Christ Community Church in Ruston, Louisiana, was kind enough to spend several hours one week helping me untangle this passage. He said, "There are dozens of Old and New Testament verses that clearly claim God does not change his mind. For example 1 Samuel 15:29 says, 'He who is the Glory of Israel does not lie or change his mind; for he is not a man, that he should change his mind.'" On the other hand, Dr. Love says that while we never have sovereignty over what God does, we are given the prerogative to influence him. "All those imperatives in Scripture don't make sense unless we can change what happens through prayer," said Love.

I was intrigued by Hezekiah's story, not only because he was healed by God after he prayed, but because his illness came after a period of high chronic stress. He was aware that the bloodthirsty Assyrians had toppled other kingdoms, and now they were at his door. Jerusalem was under siege, and Hezekiah had been humiliated in front of his people by the Assyrian leader, who taunted him and blasphemed his God. Dr. Love said, "There is no doubt that Hezekiah was under severe, life-threatening, kingdom-threatening pressure. I think having 185,000 Assyrians outside your gate—an army that had managed to subdue most of the known Middle Eastern world—would qualify one to be stressed. You can read the story in 2 Kings 18–20 and Isaiah 36–39 to get the flow of it all and the magnitude of the threat. And, yes, all of the Assyrian encounter occurred *before* his illness."

As for the king's illness, the Bible says he had a "boil." Could this have been a skin cancer, a melanoma gone wild? While I admit this is pure speculation, Deuteronomy 28:27 says, "The LORD will afflict you with the boils of Egypt and with tumors, festering sores and the itch, from which you cannot be cured." Whatever disease the king had, we know for sure that God heard his anguished prayer and not only gave him fifteen extra years but destroyed his enemies as well. How comforting to know we have a God who not only hears us when we pray but sees our tears.

After he recovered, Hezekiah reflected on his experience and concluded:

You restored me to health
and let me live.
Surely it was for my benefit
that I suffered such anguish.
In your love you kept me
from the pit of destruction;
you have put all my sins
behind your back. (Isaiah 38:16-17)

Covered by the Prayers of Others

But after we have prayed our solitary prayers, sometimes we long to hear others lovingly intone their prayers for us, and that's when we seek intercessors, those who stand before the throne of God on our behalf. John Rice, an Episcopal priest who heads Centurion House, a prayer and healing ministry in Asheville, North Carolina, regularly prays with individuals for their emotional and physical healing. "Whenever we enter God's loving presence, healing begins," says Rice, a genial man in his forties. He adds, "It's like whenever we jump into water, we get wet." Rice suggests that when we pray, God always responds, "often in the time we hope, sometimes in a different time and different way."

Rice believes that our physical and emotional well-being are anchored in the gift of salvation we receive from Jesus Christ. He told me, "I discovered that the Greek root of the word 'salvation' is *sozo,* which is also the root word for 'health,' 'wellness,' and 'wholeness.' So salvation and health are linked."

I asked him his impression of those with cancer who regularly come for prayer. Rice reflected for a moment and then said he has found that most are locked in anger, fear, bitterness, and unforgiveness. "Just as cancer eats away at the body, these negative emotions—if not dealt with—can eat away at the soul and spirit." That's why Rice believes that forgiveness—of oneself and others—is mandatory for genuine healing to occur.

Rice learned these truths at an experiential level when his mother, a director of nursing, struggled with leukemia. She experienced two remissions of cancer due not to chemotherapy, which failed to halt the progression of the disease, but to the power of prayer. On two occasions Rice, then a seminarian, flew to be with his mother to comfort her and to pray for her healing. As his mother lay in the hospital, comatose with a fever of 105 degrees, Rice felt he should not only pray for his mother's physical healing but also for "any other healing God wanted to give her." He believed his mother needed emotional healing since she and his father had experienced a crisis in their relationship when she was pregnant with John.

After the divorce, she had raised John and his sister by herself; in fact, John did not even meet his father until John was in his early thirties. So Rice prayed for the painful aftermath of a divorce that had occurred decades earlier. The next morning his mother's fever broke; she awakened and was happy and articulate. "Mother lived another year and a half after that and had a time of 'powerful testimony,'" says Rice. What about her emotional healing? Rice told me his mother asked him and his sister to forgive her for requiring their father to relinquish his visitation rights at the time of the divorce. Feeling deeply guilty, she desperately needed her children's forgiveness.

Prayer not only changes people; it changes outcomes. But what kind of prayer does Rice advocate? When people come to Centurion House for intercessory prayer, he and his team use "soaking prayer." What does he mean by this? Rice, a former agricultural extension agent, explained, "When the ground is dry, most people water it quickly, and the water runs off, failing to penetrate down to the roots. If, however, the ground is watered gently over a period of hours, then the roots are hydrated. To get to the root of our woundedness and emotional pain, we need to experience gentle, soaking prayer." To Rice, that may mean an hour a day, or even a day a week, over a period of time.

Lord, What Do You Have to Say About This Illness?

During the early days when I was praying for my own healing, a friend who had been treated for breast cancer about two years earlier challenged me not only to pray for healing but also to ask the Lord how I should view my illness. Linda Faulkner, the former social secretary for the Reagan White House, said that when her surgeon told her she had cancer and he wanted to see her the next morning, she needed to know how God viewed her illness.

"On February 27, 1995, I woke up, got dressed, and had to go before the Lord. I wanted to know what he thought about my situation. So I knelt by the bed and asked, 'Father, how am I to think about this?'" Then she started reading Jeremiah 24 and felt that God was telling her she would be healed by the "sword, famine and plague." She said that she rose from her knees ebullient, convinced she had heard from God. Never since has she been afraid of dying from cancer.

How did Linda interpret the message she believed God had given her? She admits that some may find the passage hard to relate to her situation, but she interpreted *sword* to mean surgery, *plague* to refer to chemotherapy and radiation, and *famine* to refer to the greatly improved, refined-sugar-free diet she has eaten for seven years. Faulkner told me she had been reluctant to radically change her diet until she felt the Lord told her, "I really want you to eat better." Now eight years out from her diagnosis, Linda avoids all fake, chemical foods and eats fish and organic produce whenever she can, along with fresh fruits and vegetables. She drinks vegetable juice daily. Until recently she has eaten desserts only four times a year, at holidays and on her birthday. How's that for will power?

Following my friend's advice but with some fear and trepidation, I, too, asked the Lord how I should view my illness. Was this a sickness from which I would recover? As I began reading the Bible, the words from Jeremiah 31 leapt off the page as a kind of promissory note:

I have loved you with an everlasting love;
 I have drawn you with loving-kindness.

I will build you up again
  and you will be rebuilt, O Virgin Israel.
Again you will take up your tambourines
  and go out to dance with the joyful. (verses 3-4, emphasis added)

As I read those words, I remembered the two years at London L'Abri after my first husband left me with a one-year-old and a three-year-old so he could live with the woman with whom he'd had an affair. At L'Abri the Lord rebuilt my shattered self-image, and those two years in London were a time of restoration and repair, years that helped me embrace my role as a single mother with enthusiasm and commitment, trusting God for friendships, for part-time work, for money to pay the bills, for another husband who would come along in due time and commit to me more truly than the first.

Now it seemed God was telling me he would rebuild me once again, and I sensed this meant more than just the restoration of my body. I intuited that he was to rebuild my life again—body, soul, and spirit—from the inside out.

When God Says No

But what about those who pray for healing from cancer and other diseases and die days or months or even a few short years later? When the famous Christian writer C. S. Lewis married Joy Davidman, she had metastasized breast cancer that had invaded her bones, making walking painful and difficult. As all those who have watched *Shadowlands* or read Lewis's books know, Lewis married Joy, an American citizen, after she had been diagnosed with cancer to keep her from being deported from England. Only after they married did Lewis fall in love with his wife.

After he took her to his home, the Kilns, Joy began to recover as a response to prayer, the love of her husband, and a whole new life. Her cancer went into remission for about two years, which Lewis deemed a miracle. During this period Lewis told his friend Nevill Coghill, "I never expected to have, in my sixties, the happiness that passed me by in my twenties."[12] Lewis said that he and Joy

feasted on love; every mode of it—solemn and merry, romantic and realistic,
sometimes as dramatic as a thunderstorm, sometimes as comfortable and

unemphatic as putting on your soft slippers. Her mind was as lithe and
quick and muscular as a leopard. Passion, tenderness and pain were all
equally unable to disarm it.... The most precious gift that marriage gave me
was this constant impact of something very close and intimate yet all the
while unmistakably other, resilient—in a word, real.... No cranny of heart
or body remained unsatisfied.[13]

Those famous words were written during Joy's period of remission. Sadly, it
was not to last. But even after cancer's recurrence, the couple visited Greece—Joy's
lifelong ambition—and had a splendid time. Lewis wrote a friend:

We did get to Greece, and it was a wonderful success. Joy performed prodi-
gies, climbing to the top of the Acropolis and getting as far as the Lion Gate
of Mycenae. She has (no wonder) come back very exhausted and full of
aches. But I would not have had her denied it. The condemned man is
allowed his favorite breakfast even if it is indigestible. She was absolutely
enraptured by what she saw. But pray for us: the sky grows dark.[14]

Joy died on July 12, 1960. Since then much of the world has shared in Lewis's
devastating grief recorded in the book *A Grief Observed,* which he wrote in the
days immediately following Joy's death. In this painfully honest little book,
Lewis encounters the "barrier of betrayal" and feels God has abandoned him. He
wrote:

What chokes every prayer and every hope is the memory of all the prayers
H. and I offered and all the false hopes we had. Not hopes raised merely by
our own wishful thinking; hopes encouraged, even forced upon us, by false
diagnoses, by X-ray photographs, by strange remissions, by one temporary
recovery that might have ranked as a miracle. Step by step we were "led up
the garden path." Time after time, when He seemed most gracious, He was
really preparing the next torture.[15]

The day after he wrote those words, Lewis asked, "Is it rational to believe
in a bad God? Anyway, in a God so bad as that? The Cosmic Sadist, the spiteful

imbecile?" Lewis concluded that he had projected too much errant humanity onto God, who was God, after all, and not man. He asked: "Aren't all these notes the senseless writings of a man who won't accept the fact that there is nothing we can do with suffering except to suffer it?"[16]

Fortunately, Lewis came to feel that a "locked door" no longer separated him from God. Instead, he felt that when he put his questions before God, it was as if God gazed at him in a "not uncompassionate gaze" and said, "Peace, child; you don't understand."[17] The famous Christian apologist was finally able to come to some measure of peace in recognizing that there was just too much about death and God he could not understand. He wrote, "We cannot understand. The best is perhaps what we understand least."[18]

"I Want to Soar"

Last summer when I was on grandmother duty in Chapel Hill following the birth of my second grandchild, Katie, I got word that my friend Chip Morgan had died hours after my daughter had given birth. At a time when I should have been ecstatic—I had a beautiful new granddaughter!—I was stricken that this friend had left the earth.

For about two years Chip had battled cancer, aware of the bleakness of his prognosis but at the same time solidifying his relationships with family and friends, writing for *World* magazine, hiking, traveling with his family, speaking. He also met with John Rice and his prayer team for two years and derived a great deal of hope and comfort from these weekly meetings.

Then one night I ran into him at a fund-raiser. He looked pale and physically fragile. He told me that his cancer had spread to his liver, and being a doctor, he knew his prognosis was bleak. "I may have six months left," he said. Sober but undismayed, he told those assembled that night his heartbreaking news and said that while he had never had any real assurance that God would heal the cancer, he felt the Lord had assured him he would bring glory to God as he dealt with his illness. And indeed Chip did, not only in the way he responded to cancer but in the way he touched all who crossed his path.

His wife, Becky, told me that Chip had been involved in acts of reconciliation during his battle with cancer. "Chip flew to Seattle to seek forgiveness from a high-school friend when Chip was extremely ill," she said. "He was a peacemaker. God put reconciliation in Chip's heart, and as an elder in our church, he held services of reconciliation, uniting two warring factions in our church in prayer and confession of sin."

The last time I saw Chip I went over to his home, and we sat out in the back-yard looking at the graceful sweep of his lawn, which backs up to the luxuriant Biltmore estate. "I have fourteen thousand acres here," said Chip, laughing as if he had just annexed the entire estate to his property. That day he was focused on enclosing his deck so Becky and his children could have a screened-in back porch. It was obvious he was trying to leave behind a more comfortable home for his family and that the act of doing so gave him genuine pleasure. After Chip told me about his construction plans, we talked about possible treatment for the liver cancer. He said he had decided not to take further chemo, and then this man of faith added quietly, "I am not afraid of dying." Looking at Chip that day, listening to his tone of voice, I believed him. Chip was a man at peace with himself and his God.

I don't know why Chip wasn't healed. I must admit that it temporarily rocked me that he had prayed so often and so intensely for his healing, only to leave this earth. I do know, however, he was not afraid of death, and he felt the nearness of the Lord even as his physical strength ebbed away. On Friday, the day before he died, Chip copied these verses in his journal:

Even youths grow tired and weary,
    and young men stumble and fall;
but those who hope in the LORD
    will renew their strength.
They will soar on wings like eagles;
    they will run and not grow weary,
    they will walk and not be faint. (Isaiah 40:30-31)

Underneath he wrote: "There's no thrill in walking; I want to soar." Those of us who knew this warm, honest man believe he is soaring now, even as we walk.

Folks, whether we struggle with cancer or not, we're all terminal. Earth is not our home. Since that's reality, we can confront and embrace our mortality. The best-kept secret is something the ancients knew—that it is only in facing death, our death, we finally begin to live. But even then our days are numbered, and the sum total, according to Psalm 139, God has decreed. So should we pray for healing when healing is ultimately a mystery? I believe so. We *must* pray if we truly want to live. As my friend Linda Faulkner says, "Pray for your healing until you are healed or God takes you home." That sounds good to me.

WITH A GRATEFUL HEART

Give thanks to the LORD, for he is good.
His love endures forever
PSALM 136:1

It's a guarantee that if the Lord doesn't return first, we're all going to die.
That's not a negative. That's a positive. Maintain hope in your life....
Believe that God is in control, love your family and your friends, be a
positive influence for the Lord, and lead others to the Lord.... When we
leave this world, the only thing that will go with us will be the people
who have followed Christ.

LARRY BURKETT

This past February I celebrated my sixty-second birthday with my family. As we sat around the table, savoring my favorite meal of vegetarian lasagna that my daughter Kristen had carefully prepared, a fire crackled in our stone fireplace, silver water goblets glistened in candlelight, and flowers adorned the long pine table. Amid the happy sounds of conversation, Don tapped his goblet with his spoon, and we all grew quiet. Assuming the role of master of ceremonies, my husband of twenty-eight years turned to me and asked, "Brenda, what do you wish to say to us today?"

In our family we have a birthday tradition: After the meal the honoree gets an opportunity to share birthday reflections—news from the heart. Even the children are quiet—at least reasonably so—at these moments. Knowing my time on center stage was secured, I cleared my throat and said, "My message is brief." (There was applause.) Smiling and scanning the faces of the people I love dearly, I continued, "I'm thankful to be among you today. And I'm so grateful to God that I'm alive.

The end." Katie, whose hair and face were streaked with tomato sauce, gave a gleeful squeal and rapped her spoon on her highchair tray while everyone chanted, "Hear, hear." Then Austin looked at me and said, "Mimi, you are *very* old."

It was a sweet moment and one I could not have envisioned as I reeled out of the surgeon's office six years ago, devastated by the news that I had stage 2 breast cancer and was facing even odds for survival. Each birthday postcancer I read Psalm 139 and am comforted by the words that "I am fearfully and wonderfully made" and that before I was born, the days of my life were numbered. Each birthday is a marker, a gift from the Lord, reminding me of how close I came to death and how far I've come since that cold and dark Good Friday.

Forget the wrinkles, the aging body, the thinning hair, the sun-damaged skin, and the fact that I am now old enough to qualify for Social Security. These signs of aging would have made me hysterical at fifty. But not now. Today I'm happy just to breathe, to work out at the YMCA, to travel with my husband, to write books and occasionally speak (and actually have people listen), to play with my darling grandchildren. If there's a single lesson to learn from a life-threatening disease, it is to relish the gift that is life. Today.

THE HAPPINESS QUOTIENT

Several years ago I came across an essay by Marilyn French, author of *The Women's Room* and *A Season in Hell,* a book that chronicles her battle with esophageal cancer. French states that her perspective on what constitutes happiness has changed dramatically since she developed cancer. She writes: "A serious illness or disaster is transforming. It changes not just our bodies and psyches, but the context of our desires; we choose differently, not just because we have changed but because we see different elements to choose among. For me, fresh from surviving a year's long battle with esophageal cancer, the change has been profound: My happiness quotient has changed—I am happier than I have ever been."[1]

French says that earlier in her life she was a driven woman who always lived in the future. Then her illness "shriveled the future and blew it away." She believes that losing her future was the best thing that ever happened to her because it forced her to live in the present. In the moment. In so doing, she finds her life is full of constant pleasure. She loves her work as a writer, relishes time with friends and children, and enjoys cooking "excellent food." She writes, "I move through the day from pleasure to pleasure like a woman walking through the halls of a great art gallery." The things she previously took for granted now bring her great joy. As a consequence of these internal changes, French says her laugh has changed. It's more spontaneous, deeper, richer. She ends by saying:

> I cannot say I am happy I was sick, but I am happy that sickness, if it had to happen, brought me to where I am now. It is a better place than I have ever been before. I am grateful for having been allowed to live long enough to experience it.[2]

FINAL REFLECTIONS

Like French, I believe cancer has brought me to a better place and taught me to live in the here and now. I tell people that small children, recovering alcoholics, and cancer survivors know the beauty of living in the moment. Living this way has slowed me down, changed my priorities, sweetened my relationships with friends and family, and more firmly anchored me to life than ever before. It has taught me to appreciate what I have rather than grasp for something slightly out of reach. In fact, cancer rescued me from a life "of quiet desperation." A life where I was hooked on *doing* rather than on simply *being*. A friend called this morning and at the end of our conversation told me, "Brenda, you live a far more centered, peaceful life than you did before cancer." She's right. Then I, too, was "a driven woman focused on the future" while I dragged a painful past behind me.

The beauty of cancer is that it interrupts our unbalanced, out of harmony, unfulfilling lives and confronts us head-on with the reality of our fragile mortality. It stops us in our tracks and tells us that no matter what our agenda is, we are sick, *very* sick, and our time on earth may be shorter than expected. So what are we going to do about it? Will we finally attend to the needs of our minds, bodies, and spirits? Will we solve the riddle of our painful relationships and do the work of finding something to live for that excites us and imbues each new day with a sense of meaning and purpose? Or will we keep on doing what made us sick in the first place, passively accepting our prescribed treatment without taking ownership of our disease and searching for its possible cure?

The choices are ours. But cancer is *now*. It forces its way to the top of our to-do list; in fact, it abolishes the to-do list. Confrontational, cancer asks us how we will attempt to heal our bodies and our lives—now. We may never be given a third chance; we must make the most of this second opportunity to revamp our lives and priorities. To change our perspectives on time and eternity.

For most of us, cancer is the ultimate wake-up call, causing us to totally re-evaluate our lives. Why were we created in the first place? What are we meant to do with our days on earth? In his bestseller *The Purpose-Driven Life,* Rick Warren, pastor of Saddleback Church in Lake Forest, California, states clearly that we are put "on earth to make a contribution."[3] He adds: "God wants to use you to make a difference in his world. He wants to work through you. *What matters is not the duration of your life, but the donation of it. Not how long you lived, but how you lived"* (emphasis mine).[4] Warren's point is that each of us will find the meaning and purpose we yearn for by living out our faith in Christ through serving others. And he accepts none of the excuses those of us raised in a self-aware, self-help culture have to offer:

> Abraham was old, Jacob was insecure, Leah was unattractive, Joseph was abused, Moses stuttered, Gideon was poor, Samson was codependent, Rahab was immoral, David had an affair and all kinds of family problems, Elijah was suicidal, Jeremiah was depressed, Jonah was reluctant, Naomi was a widow, John the Baptist was eccentric to say the least, Peter was impulsive and hot-tempered, Martha worried a lot, the Samaritan woman had several failed marriages, Zacchaeus was unpopular, Thomas had doubts, Paul had poor health, and Timothy was timid. That is quite a variety of misfits, but God used each of them in his service. He will use you, too, if you stop making excuses.[5]

I don't know about you, but I desire for God to use my life postcancer however he chooses. I love the verse in 1 Peter that says: "He who has suffered in his body is done with sin. As a result, he does not live the rest of his earthly life for evil human desires, but rather for the will of God" (4:1-2). Don and I pray daily that God will use us for his purposes, and we are more willing than ever to do what he requires. I've learned that sometimes he uses me when I least expect him to, in ordinary places, in nonspectacular ways.

Just this morning as I was leaving the YMCA, I had a conversation with a woman who has breast cancer. I asked how she was doing and what she was eating. She told me, "I have a hard time taking good care of myself, and I'm inconsistent with my diet. Some days I eat pretty well, and other days it's junk food all the way." And then she said, "I'm still on HRT because I don't want to go through menopause." Surprised, I asked if she was aware of the research on HRT. "No," she replied, "but I'm after quality of life, not quantity." I urged her to get a second opinion about taking HRT since she is actively battling breast cancer. "With the help of a physician who understands menopause, cancer, nutrition, and the mind-body connection, why not go for quantity of life as well as quality?" She listened and asked me for the name of a local doctor who specializes in integrative medicine.

As I got to my car, I turned to her and said, "It's all about self-love—about loving ourselves enough to become involved in our own recovery and being careful what we put into our minds and bodies."

"I think I was supposed to talk to you today," she said as she turned to go.

I then drove away, aware that I have had so many of these serendipitous conversations—phone calls from newly diagnosed cancer sufferers who are friends of friends; chance conversations at parties and gatherings; hours spent in my kitchen walking another person through my daily regimen of vitamins, juicing, and vegetarian diet; classes on nutrition I teach at church. I even had one woman come up last Sunday to tell me that before attending the class she had eaten meat and "anything with sugar." Vegetables and fruit made her ill. But she took what I said to heart and changed her diet entirely, trading meat for occasional deep-sea fish and learning to eat lots of fruits and vegetables. "I've lost thirteen pounds, and I feel so much better," she said beaming.

God is showing me daily that when he is in charge, we can touch people's lives, often in deeply meaningful ways. All we need is to be open to him and to diligently seek to do those good deeds he planned for us to do before we were even born.

I hope you are open to whatever God brings into your life from this point on and that as a result of reading this book you will do whatever it takes to try to prevent or survive cancer. I pray you will have the courage to make the strategic changes needed to give yourself the best chance of beating this disease. And never, never, never lose hope that the God who created and loves you will see you through.

I want to leave you with the words of Francis de Sales:

> Do not look forward to the changes and chances of this life in fear. Rather look at them with full hope that, as they arise, God, whose you are, will deliver you out of them. He has kept you hitherto; do you but hold fast to His dear hand, and He will lead you safely through all things; and when you cannot stand, He will bear you in His arms.
>
> Do not look forward to what may happen tomorrow. The same everlasting Father who cares for you today will take care of you tomorrow, and every day. Either He will shield you from suffering, or He will give you unfailing strength to bear it. Be at peace, then put aside all anxious thoughts and imaginations.[6]

Amen and amen. May God bless you and cherish you day by day. Whatever happens, do not give in to fear. Instead, nourish hope, love others, and press forward, savoring the day, grateful to be alive.

THE GREAT PHYSICIAN

Throughout this book I've introduced you to many distinguished physicians, two of whom have changed my life over the last six years. But I cannot end this book without telling you about the physician who has made the greatest difference in my life: Jesus Christ, the Son of God. Without his help across the years, I'm not sure I'd still be alive, enjoying friends and family and each new day. Christ has been—and continues to be—the healer of my body and the doctor of my soul.

Perhaps you are wondering how you are going to make it through this cancer zone and what is going to happen to you when you die, whether death comes in fifteen months or thirty years. You may have little confidence that your prayers are heard in heaven. You may have never read the Bible or met the Great Physician. If this is the case, I'd like to share with you how you can become acquainted with Jesus Christ and be assured of where you'll spend eternity.

Who is this Jesus? He is the Messiah, promised by God to be the Savior and deliverer of the world. He came to be a bridge between a holy God and sinful men and women. "He is the atoning sacrifice for our sins, and not only for ours but also for the sins of the whole world" (1 John 2:2). He came to set you and me free from our guilt and shame, to love us and never leave us, to fulfill our deepest yearnings for connectedness, to give us hope. To become his friend, to know him, is simple, but profound.

First, simply admit to God the obvious—that you have sinned against him, others, and yourself. In so doing, you'll agree with him about your true spiritual condition. The Bible says, "For all have sinned and fall short of the glory of God" (Romans 3:23).

Second, understand that because God is holy and because he loves you, he sent Jesus Christ, his only Son, to die an unspeakably painful death as payment for your sins and to assure your place in heaven. The Bible says, "For God so loved the world that he gave his one and only Son, that whoever believes in him shall not perish but have eternal life" (John 3:16).

Third, ask God to forgive you for all your sins and simply accept Jesus Christ as the Savior of your soul and the healer of your life. The Bible says, "If you confess with your mouth, 'Jesus is Lord,' and believe in your heart that God raised him from the dead, you will be saved" (Romans 10:9).

At this point, you may want to pray something like this: "Dear God, I know that I have sinned against you, others, and myself. I repent and am truly sorry. Forgive me for all my wrongdoings. I believe that Christ died for me, I accept his sacrifice, and I ask him to take ownership of my heart and my life from this moment forward. I am no longer my own but yours and his."

If you have sincerely prayed for Jesus to be the Lord of your life, your new life has begun. You are now a believer who will spend eternity in heaven. The Bible says, "God has given us eternal life, and this life is in his Son. He who has the Son has life; he who does not have the Son of God does not have life" (1 John 5:11-12). Moreover, you are now a new creature. "If anyone is in Christ, he is a new creation; the old has gone, the new has come!" (2 Corinthians 5:17). New attitudes. New heart. New values. New life.

Whatever happens from now on, you are not alone. You are part of that vast throng of believers who have ready access to God, the Father of all comfort, through prayer. I urge you to find a church, begin reading the Bible daily—starting with the book of John in the New Testament—and join a Bible study filled with true believers who will pray with you.

From this moment on, you have the very angels in heaven rooting for you! Not only will your present be richer and fuller, but whatever the future holds, Christ will never let you go.

And as you experience the tender care of the Father during this season of trial, you will in time be able to comfort others just as he is now comforting you. "Praise be to the God and Father of our Lord Jesus Christ, the Father of compassion and the God of all comfort, who comforts us in all our troubles, so that we can comfort those in any trouble with the comfort we ourselves have received from God" (2 Corinthians 1:3-4).

You have every reason to live, and you can face every tomorrow with joy and peace instead of fear.

NOTES

Chapter 1: Entering the Cancer Zone

1. Not his real name.
2. Not his real name.
3. John R. Lee, M.D., David Zava, and Virginia Hopkins, *What Your Doctor May Not Tell You About Breast Cancer: How Hormone Balance Can Help Save Your Life* (New York: Warner, 2002), 183.
4. Lee, Zava, and Hopkins, *What Your Doctor May Not Tell You,* 183.
5. American Cancer Society, "Cancer Facts and Figures 2003." Found at www.cancer.org on 20 May 2003.
6. Mitchell L. Gaynor and Jerry Hickey with William Fryer, *Dr. Gaynor's Cancer Prevention Program* (New York: Kensington, 1999), 7.

Chapter 2: What Is Cancer Saying About Our Lives?

1. American Cancer Society, "Cancer Facts and Figures 2003." Found at www.cancer.org on 20 May 2003.
2. American Cancer Society, "Cancer Facts and Figures 2003."
3. Geoffrey Cowley, "Now, Integrative Care," *Newsweek,* 2 December 2002, 48.
4. Cowley, "Now, Integrative Care."
5. Cowley, "Now, Integrative Care."
6. Cowley, "Now, Integrative Care."
7. W. John Diamond and W. Lee Cowden with Burton Goldberg, *An Alternative Medicine Definitive Guide to Cancer* (Tiburon, Calif.: Future Medicine, 1997), 546.
8. Diamond, Cowden, and Goldberg, *Alternative Medicine Definitive Guide,* 546.
9. Michio Kushi, *The Cancer Prevention Diet* (New York: St. Martins, 1993), 25.
10. Kushi, *The Cancer Prevention Diet.*

11. Kushi, *The Cancer Prevention Diet.*

12. M. Scott Peck, *The Road Less Traveled: A New Psychology of Love, Traditional Values, and Spiritual Growth* (New York: Simon & Schuster, 1978), 292-3.

13. Brother Lawrence, *The Practice of the Presence of God* (New York: Doubleday, 1977), 84.

14. Dr. Mitchell Gaynor, interview by author, Strang Cancer Prevention Center, New York City, 18 October 2001.

15. Lawrence L. LeShan, *Cancer As a Turning Point: A Handbook for People with Cancer, Their Families, and Health Professionals* (New York: Penguin, 1994), 13.

Chapter 3: Avoiding the Food Villains

1. Robert Marik, interview by author, 9 September 2002.

2. Mitchell L. Gaynor, M.D., "The Role of Nutrition in Cancer Prevention and Treatment," The Fifth Annual Conference in Complementary and Alternative Medicine, Duke University Program in Integrative Medicine, Durham, N.C., 18 November 2000.

3. Jean Carper, *Food—Your Miracle Medicine: How Food Can Prevent and Cure over 100 Symptoms and Problems* (San Francisco: Harper Paperbacks, 1993), 204-5.

4. Carper, *Food—Your Miracle Medicine,* 205.

5. Gaynor, "Nutrition in Cancer Prevention."

6. Unless otherwise attributed, all information from Dr. Keith Block in this chapter is taken from an interview by the author, 9 July 2003.

7. Amy O'Connor, "A Nutritional War on Cancer," *Vegetarian Times,* no. 225, May 1996, 57-8.

8. Dr. Ahmad Shamim, interview by author, 14 October 2002.

9. Patrick Quillin with Noreen Quillin, *Beating Cancer with Nutrition: Clinically Proven and Easy-to-Follow Strategies to Dramatically Improve Your Quality and Quantity of Life and Increase Chances for a Complete Remission* (Tulsa, Okla.: Nutrition Times, 1994), 122.

10. Quillin, *Beating Cancer with Nutrition.*

11. Charlotte Gerson and Morton Walker, *The Gerson Therapy: The Amazing*

Nutritional Program for Cancer and Other Illnesses (New York: Kensington, 2001), 128.

12. Quillin, *Beating Cancer with Nutrition,* 122.

13. Rex Russell, *What the Bible Says About Healthy Living: Three Biblical Principles That Will Change Your Diet and Improve Your Health* (Ventura, Calif.: Regal, 1996), 177.

14. Quillin, *Beating Cancer with Nutrition,* 122.

15. Quillin, *Beating Cancer with Nutrition,* 46.

16. Harvey Diamond and Marilyn Diamond, *Fit for Life* (New York: Warner, 1985), 105.

17. H. Diamond and M. Diamond, *Fit for Life,* 109.

18. H. Diamond and M. Diamond, *Fit for Life,* 108-9.

19. H. Diamond and M. Diamond, *Fit for Life,* 108.

20. Dr. Keith Block, quoted in Olivia Wu, "Doctor Prescribes a Regimen for Optimal Health," *Chicago Daily Herald,* 25 February 1993.

21. Russell, *What the Bible Says,* 220.

22. Dr. Keith Block, interview by author, 10 July 2003.

23. Charles B. Simone, *Cancer and Nutrition: A Ten-Point Plan to Reduce Your Risk of Getting Cancer* (Garden City Park, New York: Avery, 1992), 222.

24. H. Diamond and M. Diamond, *Fit for Life,* 111.

25. "Wendy's Loses Its Legend," *USA Today,* 9 January 2002, 1.

26. Simone, *Cancer and Nutrition,* 128-9.

27. Mitchell L. Gaynor and Jerry Hickey with William Fryer, *Dr. Gaynor's Cancer Prevention Program* (New York: Kensington, 1999), 85.

28. Dean Ornish, *Eat More, Weigh Less: Dr. Dean Ornish's Life Choice Program for Losing Weight Safely While Eating Abundantly* (San Francisco: Harper-Collins, 1993), xi.

29. Ornish, *Eat More, Weigh Less,* 30.

30. Ornish, *Eat More, Weigh Less,* 28.

31. Ellen K. Silbergeld and Polly Walker, "What If Cipro Stopped Working?" *New York Times,* 3 November 2001, op-ed, A21.

32. Silbergeld and Walker, "What If Cipro Stopped Working?" A-31.

33. Silbergeld and Walker, "What If Cipro Stopped Working?" A-31.

34. Dave Carpenter, "McDonald's Curbing Antibiotic Use in Meat," *Asheville (N.C.) Citizen Times,* 20 June 2003, B8.

35. Carper, *Food—Your Miracle Medicine,* 12-4.

36. Gaynor and Hickey with Fryer, *Dr. Gaynor's Cancer Prevention Program,* 6 (emphasis added).

Chapter 4: The Staying-Alive Diet

1. Margie Levine, *Surviving Cancer: One Woman's Story and Her Inspiring Program for Anyone Facing a Cancer Diagnosis* (New York: Broadway, 2001), 2-3.

2. Levine, *Surviving Cancer,* 9.

3. Levine, *Surviving Cancer,* 142.

4. All information from Dr. Rex Russell in this chapter is taken from an interview by the author, 16 April 2003.

5. W. John Diamond and W. Lee Cowden with Burton Goldberg, *An Alternative Medicine Definitive Guide to Cancer* (Tiburon, Calif.: Future Medicine, 1997), 568.

6. Diamond, Cowden, and Goldberg, *Alternative Medicine Definitive Guide,* 568.

7. Diamond, Cowden, and Goldberg, *Alternative Medicine Definitive Guide,* 568.

8. Diamond, Cowden, and Goldberg, *Alternative Medicine Definitive Guide,* 571-2.

9. Elizabeth Weise, "Studies Show Disturbing Amounts of Chemical Contamination in Lettuce," *USA Today,* 29 April 2003, 9D.

10. Donna L. Weihofen, "Fighting Cancer with Food and Nutrition," Complementary and Alternative Medicine Conference, Duke University and UNC Healthcare, 18 November 2000.

11. Unless otherwise attributed, all information from Dr. Keith Block in this chapter is taken from an interview by the author, 9 July 2003.

12. Jean Carper, *Food—Your Miracle Medicine: How Food Can Prevent and Cure over 100 Symptoms and Problems* (San Francisco: Harper Paperbacks, 1993), 475.

13. Janice Horowitz, "10 Foods That Pack a Wallop" *Time,* 21 January 2002, 80.

14. Carper, *Food—Your Miracle Medicine*, 480.

15. Carper, *Food—Your Miracle Medicine*, 484.

16. Carper, *Food—Your Miracle Medicine*, 487-8.

17. Donald R. Yance Jr. with Arlene Valentine, *Herbal Medicine, Healing and Cancer: A Comprehensive Program for Prevention and Treatment* (Chicago, Ill.: Keats, 1999), 65.

18. James A. Duke, "Botanical Medicine: The Amazon Experience," at the Second Annual Clinical Relevance of Medicinal Herbs and Nutritional Supplements in the Management of Major Medical Problems, University of North Carolina Schools of Medicine, Nursing, and Pharmacy, Chapel Hill, N. C., 24-26 March 2000.

19. Charlotte Gerson and Morton Walker, *The Gerson Therapy: The Amazing Nutritional Program for Cancer and Other Illnesses* (New York: Kensington, 2001), 103.

20. Mary Ruth Swope, *Green Leaves of Barley* (Phoenix: Swope Enterprises, 1987), 51.

21. Swope, *Green Leaves of Barley*, 57-8.

22. Donald O. Rudin and Clara Felix, *Omega-3 Oils: A Practical Guide* (Garden City Park, New York: Avery, 1996), 15.

23. Diamond, Cowden, and Goldberg, *Alternative Medicine Definitive Guide*, 608-10.

24. Udo Erasmus, *Fats That Heal, Fats That Kill: The Complete Guide to Fats, Oils, Cholesterol, and Human Health* (Burnaby, BC, Canada: Alive, 1993), 258-9.

25. Gerson and Walker, *The Gerson Therapy*, 98.

26. Diamond, Cowden, and Goldberg, *Alternative Medicine Definitive Guide*, 607.

27. Rex Russell, *What the Bible Says About Healthy Living* (Ventura, Calif.: Regal, 1996), 157.

28. Nick Jans, "Farmed Salmon Can't Beat Wild," *USA Today*, 7 October 2002, 12A.

29. Jans, "Farmed Salmon," 12A.

30. Marian Burros, "Farmed Salmon Looking Less Rosy," *New York Times*, 28 May, 2003, 5.

31. Burros, "Less Rosy," 5.

32. Dr. Lilian Thompson, interview by author, 7 May 2003.

33. Erasmus, *Fats That Heal,* 303.

34. Gerson and Walker, *The Gerson Therapy,* 191.

35. Horowitz, "10 Foods," 78.

36. F. Batmanghelidj, *Your Body's Many Cries for Water: You Are Not Sick, You Are Thirsty! Don't Treat Thirst with Medications* (Falls Church, Va.: Global Health Solutions, 1997), 60.

37. Batmanghelidj, *Your Body's Many Cries,* 158.

38. Batmanghelidj, *Your Body's Many Cries.* 158.

39. All the information from Dr. Dean Ornish in this chapter is taken from an interview by the author, 15 April 2003.

40. Dr. Nicholas Gonzalez, interview by author, 17 June 2002.

41. All recipes by Kelly Serbonich of Hippocrates Health Institute in West Palm Beach, Florida, are used by permission.

42. All recipes from Penny Block, *A Banquet of Health* (Evanston, Ill.: Evanston, 1994), are used with her permission.

43. All recipes from The Laughing Seed Café in Asheville, North Carolina, are used by permission.

44. All recipes from The Manatee Café in St. Augustine, Florida, are used by permission.

Chapter 5: Juicing for Life

1. Anne E. Frähm, *Cancer Battle Plan: Six Strategies for Beating Cancer from a Recovered "Hopeless Case"* (Colorado Springs: Piñon, 1992), 25.

2. Norman Walker, *Fresh Vegetable and Fruit Juices* (Prescott, Ariz.: Norwalk, 1970), 8.

3. Walker, *Fresh Vegetable and Fruit Juices,* 9.

4. Walker, *Fresh Vegetable and Fruit Juices,* 8.

5. Mitchell L. Gaynor and Jerry Hickey with William Fryer, *Dr. Gaynor's Cancer Prevention Program* (New York: Kensington, 1999), 260.

6. Charlotte Gerson and Morton Walker, *The Gerson Therapy: The Amazing Nutritional Program for Cancer and Other Illnesses* (New York: Kensington, 2001), 115.

7. Gerson and Walker, *The Gerson Therapy,* 380-1.

8. Gerson and Walker, *The Gerson Therapy,* 2.

9. Gerson and Walker, *The Gerson Therapy,* 207.

10. Gerson and Walker, *The Gerson Therapy,* 211.

11. Gerson and Walker, *The Gerson Therapy,* 200.

12. Gerson and Walker, *The Gerson Therapy,* 121-2.

13. Shared by Executive Chef Kelly Serbonich of the Hippocrates Health Institute.

Chapter 6: Detox Your Way to Health

1. Unless otherwise attributed, all the information from Dr. Nicholas Gonzalez in this chapter is taken from an interview by the author, 17 June 2002.

2. Michael Specter, "The Outlaw Doctor," *The New Yorker,* 5 February 2001, 52.

3. Specter, "The Outlaw Doctor," 52.

4. Specter, "The Outlaw Doctor," 56.

5. Charlotte Gerson and Morton Walker, *The Gerson Therapy: The Amazing Nutritional Program for Cancer and Other Illnesses* (New York: Kensington, 2001), 24-6.

6. Gerson and Walker, *The Gerson Therapy,* 30.

7. Gerson and Walker, *The Gerson Therapy,* 31-2.

8. Gerson and Walker, *The Gerson Therapy,* 44.

9. W. John Diamond and W. Lee Cowden with Burton Goldberg, *An Alternative Medicine Definitive Guide to Cancer* (Tiburon, Calif.: Future Medicine, 1997), 188.

10. Gerson and Walker, *The Gerson Therapy,* 207.

11. Gerson and Walker, *The Gerson Therapy,* 211.

Chapter 7: Nurturing Ourselves—Selfish or Self-Preservation?

1. Alice D. Domar, "The Healing Art of Self-Nurturance" at the Women, Wellness and the Transformation of Health Care Conference, Duke Center for Integrative Medicine, Durham, N.C., 12 October 2002.

2. Domar, "The Healing Art of Self-Nurturance."

3. Randy Peyser, "Health and Spirituality," *Alternative Medicine,* April 2002, 108.

4. Peyser, "Health and Spirituality," 106.

5. Peyser, "Health and Spirituality," 110.

6. Caryle Hirshberg and Marc Ian Barasch, *Remarkable Recovery: What Extraordinary Healings Tell Us About Getting Well and Staying Well* (New York: Riverhead, 1995), 165.

7. Hirshberg and Barasch, *Remarkable Recovery,* 165-6.

8. Hirshberg and Barasch, *Remarkable Recovery,* 168-9.

9. Domar, "The Healing Art of Self-Nurturance."

10. W. John Diamond and W. Lee Cowden with Burton Goldberg, *An Alternative Medicine Definitive Guide to Cancer* (Tiburon, Calif.: Future Medicine, 1997), 295.

11. Diamond, Cowden, and Goldberg, *Alternative Medicine Definitive Guide,* 631.

12. Diamond, Cowden, and Goldberg, *Alternative Medicine Definitive Guide,* 631.

13. Diamond, Cowden, and Goldberg, *Alternative Medicine Definitive Guide,* 631.

14. Diamond, Cowden, and Goldberg, *Alternative Medicine Definitive Guide,* 76.

15. Diamond, Cowden, and Goldberg, *Alternative Medicine Definitive Guide,* 296.

16. Diamond, Cowden, and Goldberg, *Alternative Medicine Definitive Guide,* 1003.

17. Lorraine Day, *You Can't Improve on God,* 92 min., Rockford Press, 1997, videocassette. You can contact Rockford Press at P. O. Box 8, Thousand Palms, CA 92286 or at 1-800-574-2437.

18. Christine Gorman, "Walk, Don't Run," *Time,* 21 January 2002, 82.

19. Ann Japenga, "Strong Woman," *Health,* November-December 1999, 136-46.

20. Japenga, "Strong Woman," 146.

21. Ruth Heidrich, *A Race for Life: A Diet and Exercise Program for Superfitness and Reversing the Aging Process: The Amazing Story of How One Woman Survived Breast Cancer to Take on the Toughest Races in the World* (New York: Lantern, 2000), 148.

22. Heidrich, *A Race for Life,* 149.

23. Donald R. Yance Jr. with Arlene Valentine, *Herbal Medicine, Healing and Cancer: A Comprehensive Program for Prevention and Treatment* (Chicago, Ill.: Keats, 1999), 259.

24. Yance Jr. and Valentine, *Herbal Medicine,* 259.

25. Yance Jr. and Valentine, *Herbal Medicine,* 260.

26. Day, *You Can't Improve on God.*

27. Yance Jr. and Valentine, *Herbal Medicine,* 259.

28. Yance Jr. and Valentine, *Herbal Medicine,* 259.

29. Yance Jr. and Valentine, *Herbal Medicine,* 261.

30. Dr. Mitchell Gaynor, interview by author, 18 October 2001.

31. Mitchell L. Gaynor, *The Healing Power of Sound: A Physician Reveals the Therapeutic Power of Sound, Voice, and Music* (Boston: Shambhala, 2002), 82-3.

32. Gaynor, *The Healing Power of Sound,* 82-3.

33. Philip Yancey and Tim Stafford, "Lyrics for the Living God," *The Student Bible, New International Version* (Grand Rapids, Mich.: Zondervan, 1996), 592.

34. Herbert Benson, *The Relaxation Response* (New York: HarperCollins, 1975), 10.

35. Herbert Benson with William Proctor, *Beyond the Relaxation Response: How to Harness the Healing Power of Your Personal Beliefs* (New York: Berkeley, 1984), 107.

36. Stephanie Kirch, "Cancer: Tests Showed No Growth in Tumor," *Asheville (N. C.) Citizen Times,* 30 October 2000.

Chapter 8: A Healing Place

1. Names of many of the guests have been changed to protect their identities.

2. *Hippocrates News,* vol. 17, no. 3, 1998.

3. Harvey Diamond and Marilyn Diamond, *Fit for Life* (New York: Warner, 1985), 65.

Chapter 9: The Will to Live

1. John 5:6.

2. John 5:7.

3. John 5:8.

4. Norman Cousins, *Anatomy of an Illness as Perceived by the Patient: Reflections on Healing and Regeneration* (New York: Bantam, 1979), 31.

5. Cousins, *Anatomy of an Illness*, 31.

6. Cousins, *Anatomy of an Illness*, 29.

7. Cousins, *Anatomy of an Illness*, 40.

8. Cousins, *Anatomy of an Illness*, 45 (emphasis added).

9. Lawrence L. LeShan, *Cancer As a Turning Point: A Handbook for People with Cancer, Their Families, and Health Professionals* (New York: Penguin, 1994), xii.

10. LeShan, *Cancer As a Turning Point*, 113 (emphasis added).

11. LeShan, *Cancer As a Turning Point*, 114.

12. LeShan, *Cancer As a Turning Point*, 117.

13. LeShan, *Cancer As a Turning Point*, 3.

14. LeShan, *Cancer As a Turning Point*, 3.

15. Dr. Ruth Bollentino, interview by author, 17 October 2001.

16. Sir James Paget, *Surgical Pathology* (London: Longman, Brown, Green, and Longmans, 1853), quoted in LeShan, *Cancer As a Turning Point*, 10.

17. LeShan, *Cancer As a Turning Point*, 14.

18. LeShan, *Cancer As a Turning Point*, 15.

19. Linda Seligman, *Promoting a Fighting Spirit: Psychotherapy for Cancer Patients, Survivors, and Their Families* (San Francisco: Jossey-Bass, 1996), 9.

20. Seligman, *Promoting a Fighting Spirit*, 9-10.

21. Dr. James Gordon, interview by author, Strang Cancer Institute, 1 November 2002.

22. Bollentino interview.

23. Dr. Mitchell Gaynor, interview by author, 18 October 2001.

24. Robert Browning, "Rabbi Ben Ezra" as quoted in *The Literature of England: An Anthology and History,* single volume edition (Chicago: Scott, Foresman and Company, 1953), 879.

Chapter 10: Chronic Stress and Cancer

1. Larry Burkett, interview by author, 25 April 2003.

2. *Harvard Mental Health Letter,* 1 April 2002.

3. Robert M. Sapolsky, *Why Zebras Don't Get Ulcers: An Updated Guide to Stress, Stress-Related Diseases, and Coping* (New York: W. H. Freeman, 1998), 6.

4. Sapolsky, *Why Zebras Don't Get Ulcers,* 10.

5. Sapolsky, *Why Zebras Don't Get Ulcers,* 10-1.

6. Sapolsky, *Why Zebras Don't Get Ulcers,* 135-6.

7. Sapolsky, *Why Zebras Don't Get Ulcers,* 133-4.

8. Sapolsky, *Why Zebras Don't Get Ulcers,* 132-3.

9. David Spiegel et al., "Effects of Psychosocial Treatment in Prolonging Cancer Survival May Be Mediated by Neuroimmune Pathways," *Annals of the New York Academy of Sciences* 840 (1998): 674-83.

10. Spiegel, "Effects of Psychosocial Treatment."

11. Dr. Bob Maunder, interview by author, 6 October 2002.

12. C. Maddock and C. M. Pariante, "How Does Stress Affect You? An Overview of Immunity, Depression and Disease," *Epidemiology, Psychiatry and Sociology* 10, no. 3 (July-September 2001): 153-62.

13. Maunder interview.

14. C. C. Chen et al., "Adverse Life Events and Breast Cancer: Case Controlled Study," *British Medical Journal* (9 December 1995): 1527-30.

15. A. J. Ramirez et al., "Stress and Relapse of Breast Cancer," *British Medical Journal* (4 February 1989): 1032.

16. Erica Goode, "The Heavy Cost of Chronic Stress," *New York Times,* 17 December 2002, 17.

17. Lydia R. Temoshok, "Connecting the Dots Linking Mind, Behavior, Disease: The Biological Concomitants of Coping Patterns: Commentary on 'Attachment and Cancer: A Conceptual Integration,'" *Integrative Medicine Therapies* 1, no. 4 (2002): 387.

18. Temoshok, "Connecting the Dots," 387.

19. Goode, "Cost of Chronic Stress," 17.

20. C. M. Fox et al., "Loneliness, Emotional Repression, Marital Quality and Major Life Events in Women Who Develop Breast Cancer," *Journal of Community Health* 6 (19 December 1994): 467-82.

21. Marilyn Elias, "Study Suggests Stress Before Cancer Diagnosis Can Raise Death Risk," *USA Today,* 11 March 2003, 10D.

22. Donald Yance, "Assessing and Treating Adrenal and Thyroid Deficient

Disorders," *Official Proceedings,* Medicines from the Earth Conference, Asheville, N. C., June 2002, 153.

23. Burkett interview.

24. Rick Lavender, "Larry Burkett: His Christian View of Finances Touched People Around the World," *Gainesville (Georgia) Times,* 6 July 2003, front page.

Chapter 11: Emotions and Cancer

1. Alice Hopper Epstein, *Mind, Fantasy and Healing: One Woman's Journey from Conflict and Illness to Wholeness and Health* (New York: Delacorte, 1989), 49-50.

2. Epstein, *Mind, Fantasy and Healing,* 50.

3. Epstein, *Mind, Fantasy and Healing,* xxi.

4. Epstein, *Mind, Fantasy and Healing,* xxii.

5. Alice Epstein, telephone conversation with author, 17 September 2002.

6. Seymour Epstein, telephone conversation with author, 17 September 2002.

7. Lawrence L. LeShan, *Cancer As a Turning Point: A Handbook for People with Cancer, Their Families, and Health Professionals* (New York: Penguin, 1994), 10.

8. Sir James Paget, *Surgical Pathology* (London: Longman, Brown, Green, and Longmans, 1853), quoted in LeShan, *Cancer As a Turning Point,* 10.

9. W. John Diamond and W. Lee Cowden with Burton Goldberg, *An Alternative Medicine Definitive Guide to Cancer* (Tiburon, Calif.: Future Medicine, 1997), 617.

10. Candace Pert, *Molecules of Emotion* (New York: Scribner, 1997), quoted in Bill Moyers, *Healing and the Mind* (New York: Doubleday, 1993), 183.

11. Pert, *Molecules,* quoted in Moyers, *Healing and the Mind,* 189.

12. Candace Pert, Henry Dreher, Michael Ruff, "The Psychosomatic Network: Foundations of Mind-Body Medicine," *Alternative Therapies* 4, no. 4 (July 1998): 31.

13. Pert, *Molecules,* quoted in Moyers, *Healing and the Mind,* 191.

14. Diamond, Cowden, and Goldberg, *Alternative Medicine Definitive Guide,* 617.

15. Diamond, Cowden, and Goldberg, *Alternative Medicine Definitive Guide,* 617.

16. Pert, Dreher, and Ruff, "The Psychosomatic Network," 36.

17. Pert, Dreher, and Ruff, "The Psychosomatic Network," 36 (emphasis added).

18. Sigmund Freud, *Outline of Psychoanalysis* (London: Hogarth, 1940), 188.

19. Larry Burkett, telephone conversation with author, 25 April 2003.

20. Dr. James Gordon, interview by author, 1 November 2002.

21. Dr. Lydia Temoshok, interview by author, 13 March 2003.

22. Marabel Morgan, interview by author, 15 October 2002.

23. Dr. Gonzalez, interview by author, 17 June 2002.

Chapter 12: Why We Need Our Friends—and Others

1. Robert Bell, *Worlds of Friendship* (Beverly Hills, Calif.: Sage, 1981), 65.

2. Margie Levine, *Surviving Cancer: One Woman's Story and Her Inspiring Program for Anyone Facing a Cancer Diagnosis* (New York: Broadway, 2001), 75.

3. Alice D. Domar, "The Healing Art of Self-Nurturance" at the Women, Wellness and the Transformation of Health Care Conference, Duke Center for Integrative Medicine, Durham, N.C., 12 October 2002.

4. Ina Yalof, ed., *Straight from the Heart: Letters of Hope and Inspiration from Survivors of Breast Cancer* (New York: Kensington, 1996), 26.

5. Yalof, *Straight from the Heart,* 133.

6. Linda Seligman, *Promoting a Fighting Spirit: Psychotherapy for Cancer Patients, Survivors, and Their Families* (San Francisco: Jossey-Bass, 1996), 162.

7. David Spiegel, "Effects of Psychosocial Support on Patients with Metastatic Breast Cancer," *Journal of Psychosocial Oncology* 10, no. 2 (1992): 113-20.

8. F. I. Fawzy et al., "Malignant Melanoma: Effects of an Early Structured Psychiatric Intervention, Coping and Affective State on Recurrence and Survival Six Years Later," *Archives of General Psychiatry* 50, no. 9 (1993): 681-9.

9. Alastair J. Cunningham, *Beginning Your Healing Journey Workbook* (Toronto, Ontario, Canada: World Health Services Council, 2001), 22.

10. Cunningham, *Beginning Your Healing,* 22.

11. All the information from Dr. Shirley Taffel in this chapter was taken from an interview by the author, 11 April 2003.

Chapter 13: Dealing with Difficult People

1. Dean Ornish, *Love and Survival: The Scientific Basis for the Healing Power of Intimacy* (New York: HarperCollins, 1998), 37.
2. Ornish, *Love and Survival*, 62.
3. Ornish, *Love and Survival*, 63.
4. Ornish, *Love and Survival*, 63.
5. Linda Seligman, *Promoting a Fighting Spirit: Psychotherapy for Cancer Patients, Survivors, and Their Families* (San Francisco: Jossey-Bass, 1996), 184.
6. Harold Bloomfield with Philip Goldberg, *Making Peace with Your Past: The Six Essential Steps to Enjoying a Great Future* (New York: HarperCollins, 2000), 187.
7. Bloomfield with Goldberg, *Making Peace with Your Past*, 187.
8. Henry Cloud and John Townsend, *How People Grow: What the Bible Reveals About Personal Growth* (Grand Rapids: Zondervan, 2001), 180.
9. Cloud and Townsend, *How People Grow*, 180.
10. Bloomfield with Goldberg, *Making Peace with Your Past*, 193.
11. C. S. Lewis, *Letters to an American Lady*, ed. Clyde S. Kilby (London, England: Hodder and Stoughton, 1967), 92.
12. Lewis, *Letters to an American Lady*, 93.
13. Lewis, *Letters to an American Lady*, 117.
14. Lewis, *Letters to an American Lady*, 117.
15. Dr. Gonzalez, interview by author, 17 June 2002.

Chapter 14: Embracing Life

1. Lawrence L. LeShan, *Cancer As a Turning Point: A Handbook for People with Cancer, Their Families, and Health Professionals* (New York: Penguin, 1994), 23.
2. LeShan, *Cancer As a Turning Point*, 23.
3. LeShan, *Cancer As a Turning Point*, 43.
4. LeShan, *Cancer As a Turning Point*, 32-5.
5. Dr. Gary Cobb, interview by author, 16 October 2002.
6. Geri Blair, "Faith and Attitude," *Coping*, July-August 1998, 34.

7. Blair, "Faith and Attitude," 34.

8. LeShan, *Cancer As a Turning Point,* 72-3.

9. LeShan, *Cancer As a Turning Point,* 73.

Chapter 15: The Healing Power of Faith

1. David Jeremiah, "A Story of Cancer and Comfort," part 2, interview by James Dobson, *Focus on the Family,* 3 June 2002.

2. David Jeremiah, interview by author, 30 October 2002.

3. Jeremiah, "A Story of Cancer."

4. Jeremiah, "A Story of Cancer."

5. Dr. Harold Koenig, interview by author, 20 September 2002.

6. Koenig interview.

7. Harold G. Koenig, *The Healing Power of Faith: Science Explores Medicine's Last Great Frontier* (New York: Simon and Schuster, 1999), 24.

8. Koenig, *The Healing Power of Faith,* 24.

9. Koenig, *The Healing Power of Faith,* 25.

10. Rex Russell, *What the Bible Says About Healthy Living: Three Biblical Principles That Will Change Your Diet and Improve Your Health* (Ventura, Calif.: Regal, 1996), 20.

11. Russell, *What the Bible Says,* 37 (emphasis added).

12. Roger Lancelyn Green and Walter Hooper, *C .S. Lewis: A Biography* (London: St. James Place, 1974), 270.

13. Green and Hooper, *C .S. Lewis,* 277-8.

14. C. S. Lewis, *Letters to an American Lady,* ed. Clyde. S. Kilby (England: Hodder and Stoughton, 1967), 88.

15. C. S. Lewis, *A Grief Observed* (New York: Harper & Row, 1961), 26-7.

16. Lewis, *A Grief Observed,* 29.

17. Lewis, *A Grief Observed,* 54.

18. Lewis, *A Grief Observed,* 59.

Chapter 16: With a Grateful Heart

1. Marilyn French, "My Happiness Quotient," *Family Circle,* 1 February 1999, 122.

2. French, "My Happiness Quotient," 122.

3. Rick Warren, *The Purpose-Driven Life* (Grand Rapids: Zondervan, 2002), 227.

4. Warren, *The Purpose-Driven Life,* 233.

5. Warren, *The Purpose-Driven Life,* 233.

6. Francis de Sales, quoted in Mrs. Charles E. Cowman, comp., *Streams in the Desert* (1925; repr., Grand Rapids: Zondervan, 1965), 51.